Study Guide
Cooper & Gosnell

Adult Health Nursing

Seventh Edition

Candice Kumagai

Formerly Instructor in Clinical Nursing
University of Texas at Austin
Austin, Texas

ELSEVIER
MOSBY

ELSEVIER
MOSBY

3251 Riverport Lane
St. Louis, Missouri 63043

STUDY GUIDE FOR ADULT HEALTH NURSING, Seventh edition   ISBN: 978-0-323-11221-5

Content Strategist: Nancy O'Brien
Content Development Specialist: Kelly Skelton
Publishing Services Manager: Jeff Patterson
Project Manager: Mary G. Stueck
Design Direction: Karen Pauls

Printed in Canada

Last digit is the print number: 9 8 7 6 5 4 3 2 1

To the Student

Understanding fundamental concepts and principles of medical-surgical nursing will prepare you for patient care experiences. By mastering the content of your *Adult Health Nursing* textbook, you will have the necessary knowledge and skills for nursing practice. This Study Guide was created to help you achieve the objectives of each chapter in the textbook, establish a solid base of knowledge in the fundamentals of nursing, and evaluate your understanding of this critical information.

Each Study Guide chapter is organized into sections, each with its own topic and related objectives from the textbook. Different types of learning activities, including short answer, multiple choice, fill-in-the blank, matching, and true/false, assist you in meeting these content objectives. To maximize the benefits of this Study Guide and prepare for the learning activities:

1. Carefully read the chapter in the textbook and highlight, note, or outline important information.
2. Review the Key Points, access the Additional Learning Resources, and complete the Review Questions for the NCLEX® Examination at the end of each textbook chapter.
3. Complete the Study Guide exercises to the best of your ability.
4. Time and pace yourself during the completion of each exercise. You should spend approximately 1 minute for each multiple choice, true/false, and matching question, and approximately 2 minutes for completion activities or short answer questions.
5. After completing an exercise, refer to the textbook page references as needed. You can then repeat any exercises for additional practice and review. A complete Answer Key is provided in your Additional Learning Resources on Evolve.

ADDITIONAL LEARNING RESOURCES

Additional Learning Resources are available on the Evolve website at http://evolve.elsevier.com/Cooper/adult.

Evolve

- Review Questions for the NCLEX® Examination (for each chapter)
- Answer Key for all Study Guide questions
- Calculators
- Additional Animations
- Additional Video Clips
- Additional Audio Clips
- Skills Performance Checklists
- Spanish/English Glossary
- Body Spectrum Electronic Anatomy Coloring Book
- Fluid and Electrolytes Tutorial

STUDY HINTS FOR ALL STUDENTS

- *Ask questions!* There are no bad questions. If you do not know something or are not sure, you need to find out. Other people may be wondering the same thing but may be too shy to ask. The answer could mean life or death to your patient, which certainly is more important than feeling embarrassed about asking a question.

- *Make use of chapter objectives.* At the beginning of each chapter in the textbook are objectives that you should have mastered when you finish studying that chapter. Write these objectives in your notebook, leaving a blank space after each. Fill in the answers as you find them while reading the chapter. Review to make sure your answers are correct and complete, and use these answers when you study for tests. This should also be done for separate course objectives that your instructor has listed in your class syllabus.
- *Locate and understand key terms.* At the beginning of each chapter in the textbook are key terms that you will encounter as you read the chapter. Page numbers are provided for easy reference and review, and the key terms are in bold, blue font the first time they appear in the chapter. Phonetic pronunciations are provided for terms that might be difficult to pronounce.
- *Review Key Points.* Use the Key Points at the end of each chapter in the textbook to help you review for exams.
- *Get the most from your textbook.* When reading each chapter in the textbook, look at the subject headings to learn what each section is about. Read first for the general meaning, then reread parts you did not understand. It may help to read those parts aloud. Carefully read the information given in each table and study each figure and its caption.
- *Follow up on difficult concepts.* While studying, put difficult concepts into your own words to see if you understand them. Check this understanding with another student or the instructor. Write these in your notebook.
- *Take useful notes.* When taking lecture notes in class, leave a large margin on the left side of each notebook page and write only on right-hand pages, leaving all left-hand pages blank. Look over your lecture notes soon after each class, while your memory is fresh. Fill in missing words, complete sentences and ideas, and underline key phrases, definitions, and concepts. At the top of each page, write the topic of that page. In the left margin, write the key word for that part of your notes. On the opposite left-hand page, write a summary or outline that combines material from both the textbook and the lecture. These can be your study notes for review.
- *Join or form a study group.* Form a study group with some other students so you can help one another. Practice speaking and reading aloud, ask questions about material you are not sure about, and work together to find answers.
- *Improve your study skills.* Good study skills are essential for achieving your goals in nursing. Time management, efficient use of study time, and a consistent approach to studying are all beneficial. There are various study methods for reading a textbook and for taking class notes. Some methods that have proven helpful can be found in *Saunders Student Nurse Planner: A Guide to Success in Nursing School* by Susan C. deWit. This book contains helpful information on test-taking and preparing for clinical experiences. It includes an example of a "time map" for planning study time and a blank form that you can use to formulate a personal time map.

ADDITIONAL STUDY HINTS FOR STUDENTS WHO USE ENGLISH AS A SECOND LANGUAGE (ESL)

- *Find a first-language buddy.* ESL students should find a first-language buddy—another student who is a native speaker of English and is willing to answer questions about word meanings, pronunciations, and culture. Maybe your buddy would like to learn about your language and culture. This could help in his or her nursing experience as well.
- *Expand your vocabulary.* If you find a nontechnical word you do not know (e.g., *drowsy*), try to guess its meaning from the sentence (e.g., *With electrolyte imbalance, the patient may feel fatigued and drowsy*). If you are not sure of the meaning, or if it seems particularly important, look it up in the dictionary.
- *Keep a vocabulary notebook.* Keep a small alphabetized notebook or address book in which you can write down new nontechnical words you read or hear along with their meanings and pronunciations. Write each word under its initial letter so you can find it easily, as in a dictionary. For words you do not know or for words that have a different meaning in nursing, write down how they are used and sound. Look up their meanings in a dictionary or ask your instructor or first-

language buddy. Then write the different meanings or usages that you have found in your book, including the nursing meaning. Continue to add new words as you discover them. For example:

- *Primary*—Of most importance; main (e.g., *the primary problem or disease*); The first one; elementary (e.g., *primary school*)
- *Secondary*—Of less importance; resulting from another problem or disease (e.g., *a secondary symptom*); The second one (e.g., *secondary school ["high school" in the United States]*)

Illustration Credits

Chapter 1

P. 3: Harkreader H, Hogan MA, & Thobaben M: *Fundamentals of nursing: Caring and clinical judgment*, ed 3, St. Louis, 2007, Saunders.

Chapter 3

P. 17: Thibodeau GA & Patton KT: *Anthony's textbook of anatomy and physiology*, ed 20, St. Louis, 2013, Mosby.

Chapter 4

P. 21: Patton KT & Thibodeau GA: *The human body in health and disease*, ed 6, St. Louis, 2014, Mosby.

Chapter 5

P. 27: Thibodeau GA & Patton KT: *Anatomy and physiology*, ed 8, St. Louis, 2013, Mosby.

Chapter 8

P. 48: Canobbio M: *Mosby's clinical nursing series: Cardiovascular disorders*, St. Louis, 1990, Mosby.

Chapter 11

P. 74: Patton KT & Thibodeau GA: *Anatomy and physiology*, ed 8, St. Louis, 2013, Mosby.

Chapter 12

P. 81: Patton KT & Thibodeau GA: *The human body in health and disease*, ed 6, St. Louis, 2014, Mosby.

P. 84: Seidel HM, Ball JW, Dains JE, et al.: *Mosby's guide to physical examination*, ed 7, St. Louis, 2011, Mosby.

Chapter 13

P. 91: Thibodeau GA & Patton KT: *Structure and function of the body*, ed 14, St. Louis, 2012, Mosby.

P. 94: Thibodeau GA & Patton KT: *Anthony's textbook of anatomy and physiology*, ed 20, St. Louis, 2013, Mosby.

Chapter 14

P. 101: Thibodeau GA & Patton KT: *Structure and function of the body*, ed 14, St. Louis, 2012, Mosby.

P. 103: Ignatavicius DD & Workman ML: *Medical-surgical nursing: Patient-centered collaborative care*, ed 6, St. Louis, 2010, Saunders.

Chapter 15

P. 109: Grimes D: *Infectious diseases*, St. Louis, 1991, Mosby.

Introduction to Anatomy and Physiology

chapter

1

Answer Key: Textbook page references are provided as a guide for answering these questions. A complete Answer Key is provided in your Additional Learning Resources on Evolve.

CROSSWORD PUZZLE

1. Directions: Use the clues to complete the crossword puzzle.

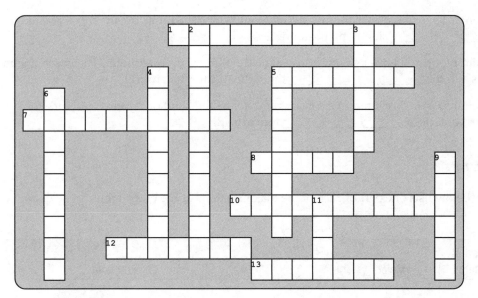

Across

1. Engulf and digest foreign material *(7)*
5. Cell division *(6)*
7. Movement of water and particles through a membrane by force from either pressure or gravity *(8)*
8. Several kinds of tissues united to perform a more complex function *(11)*
10. Extracellular fluid taken into the cell and digested *(7)*
12. Diffusion of water through a selectively permeable membrane in the presence of at least one impermeant solute *(8)*
13. Largest organelle within the cell *(5)*

Down

2. Body's internal environment is relatively constant *(5)*
3. Perform more complex functions than any one organ can perform alone *(11)*
4. Internal living material of cells *(5)*
5. Thin sheets of tissue that serve many functions in the body *(5)*
6. Solid particles in a fluid move from an area of higher concentration to an area of lower concentration *(7)*
9. Groups of similar cells that work together to perform a specific function *(9)*
11. Smallest living unit of structure and function in the body *(4)*

FILL-IN-THE-BLANK SENTENCES

Directions: Complete each sentence by filling in the blank with the correct terminology that the nurse uses to document and identify location on the human body.

2. The patient reports, "I ran into the coffeetable and bruised my shin." Nurse documents: 4-cm area of ecchymosis noted on the mid-_____ of right lower extremity. *(1)*

3. The patient reports, "I was laying on my stomach, so my entire back got sunburned." Nurse documents: Superficial sunburn sustained on _____ body surface. *(1)*

4. The patient states, "I have small lump just above my collarbone." Nurse documents: 3-cm nontender nodule _____ to the midclavicular area. *(1)*

5. After being in an automobile accident, the patient has many abrasions on the surface of the skin. Nurse documents: Multiple _____ lacerations. *(2)*

6. The patient states, "I noticed a patch of dry, itchy skin just underneath my bellybutton." Nurse documents: 4-cm dry, scaly skin _____ to umbilicus. *(1)*

7. The patient reports, "Occasionally I have a mild pain in the middle of my chest." The nurse documents: Occasional mild pain in the _____ chest area. *(1)*

8. The patient asks for assistance to turn onto the right side. The nurse documents: Assisted into a right _____ side-lying position. *(1)*

9. The patient reports, "I have lost sensation in the tip of my right ring finger. The nurse documents: Paresthesia in the _____ tip of the fourth phalanx. *(2)*

10. The patient reports, "My forearm is tender right below the bend of my elbow." Nurse documents: Tenderness anterior _____ forearm. *(2)*

TABLE ACTIVITY

11. The table below lists one part of each of the major systems of the body. Identify the major system and then identify at least one function. *(12)*

One Body Part of Major System	Major System	Function
Lungs		
Heart		
Brain		
Stomach		
Kidneys		
Bones		
Voluntary muscles		
Skin		
Thyroid gland		
Lymph nodes		
Gonads		

FIGURE LABELING

Planes of the Body

12. Directions: Label the figure below with the correct names of the body planes and anatomical directionality of the body: sagittal; coronal, ventral, dorsal, transverse, caudal, and cranial. *(2)*

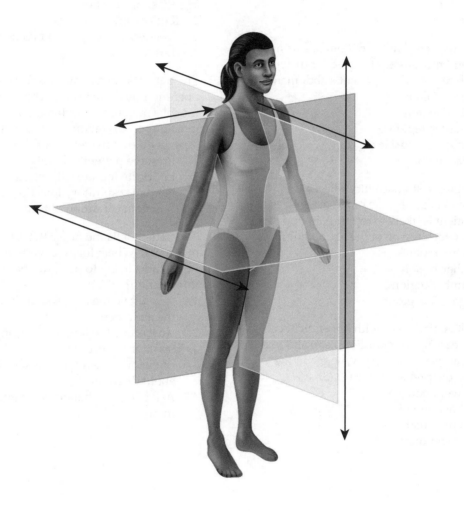

MULTIPLE CHOICE

Directions: Select the best answer(s) for each of the following questions.

13. The patient reports pain in the right upper abdomen just inferior to the ribs. Based on the nurse's knowledge of anatomy, which organ is most likely to be contributing to the patient's discomfort? *(3)*
    1. Small intestine
    2. Spleen
    3. Gallbladder
    4. Cecum

14. The nurse suspects that the patient has urinary retention and must assess for bladder distention. Which region of the patient's abdomen will the nurse palpate? *(3)*
    1. Umbilical region
    2. Hypogastric region
    3. Right hypochondriac region
    4. Left iliac region

15. The patient has a stomach ulcer. Based on knowledge of anatomy, the nurse recognizes that the patient is likely to report pain or discomfort in which region of the abdomen? *(3)*
    1. Epigastric region
    2. Right iliac region
    3. Left lumbar region
    4. Hypogastric region

16. The patient is diagnosed with appendicitis. The health care provider orders ice to abdomen pending emergency surgery. Where will the nurse place the prepared icebag? *(3)*
    1. Left lower quadrant
    2. Right lower quadrant
    3. Left upper quadrant
    4. Right upper quadrant

17. In the case of bowel obstruction, which condition is most likely to cause the first episodes of vomiting if the patient is allowed to consume solid foods? *(1)*
    1. Distal large intestine obstruction
    2. Proximal large intestine obstruction
    3. Distal small intestine obstruction
    4. Proximal small intestine obstruction

18. The patient sustains injury to the epidermis. Which problem will the nurse anticipate and try to prevent? *(10)*
    1. Risk for infection
    2. Loss of strength
    3. Decreased secretion of mucus
    4. Loss of insulation

19. The patient is in a coma and has continuous open-mouthed breathing, which causes dry mucous membranes of the mouth. What is the most important rationale for the nurse to perform good oral hygiene for this patient? *(11)*
    1. Preserve patient's dignity
    2. Lubricate food for digestion
    3. Prevent respiratory infection
    4. Maintain condition of teeth

20. The patient tells the nurse that he has a history of bursitis. Which focused assessment is the nurse most likely to perform that relates to this information? *(11)*
    1. Auscultate the bowel sounds and palpate the abdomen
    2. Auscultate the lung sounds and watch respiratory effort
    3. Put joints through range of motion and ask about discomfort
    4. Ask patient to balance on right leg and then on left leg

CRITICAL THINKING ACTIVITIES

Activity 1

21. Why is it important for the nurse to have knowledge of anatomy and physiology? *(1)*

_____

_____

_____

Activity 2

22. The patient says, "I have a bruise on the tip of my right big toe." Document the patient's report using anatomical terminology. *(1)*

_____

Activity 3

23. Discuss how the accurate usage and correct spelling of anatomical terminology enhances the credibility of your nursing documentation. *(1)*

_____

_____

_____

Care of the Surgical Patient

Answer Key: Textbook page references are provided as a guide for answering these questions. A complete Answer Key is provided in your Additional Learning Resources on Evolve.

MATCHING

Directions: Match the term or suffix on the left with the meaning on the right. (16)

		Term		**Meaning**
_____	1.	anastomosis	a.	Surgical removal of
			b.	Direct visualization by a scope
_____	2.	-ectomy	c.	Opening into
_____	3.	-lysis	d.	Surgical joining of two ducts or blood vessels to allow flow from one to another; to bypass an area
_____	4.	-orrhaphy	e.	Surgical repair of
_____	5.	-oscopy	f.	Destruction or dissolution of
_____	6.	-ostomy	g.	Opening made to allow the passage of drainage
			h.	Plastic surgery
_____	7.	-otomy	i.	Fixation of
_____	8.	-pexy		
_____	9.	-plasty		

TRUE OR FALSE

Directions: Write T for true or F for false in the blanks provided. (16)

_____ 10. A rhinoplasty could be performed for cosmetic reasons.

_____ 11. Removal of the appendix is an ablative type of surgery.

_____ 12. A breast biopsy is a palliative surgery.

_____ 13. The surgeon may perform an exploratory laparotomy to confirm a diagnosis.

_____ 14. A carotid endarterectomy could be performed under same-day admit conditions.

_____ 15. Total hip replacement is a type of transplant surgery.

_____ 16. Closure of an atrial septal defect in the heart is constructive surgery.

_____ 17. Internal fixation of a right fibula is reconstructive surgery.

_____ 18. Coronary artery bypass is one example of major surgery.

_____ 19. Cataract extraction is usually considered an urgent surgery.

TABLE ACTIVITY

20. Directions: The patient has just returned from gastric surgery. Next to each assessment, list what normal findings the nurse would expect and how frequently the data collection would be performed. *(44-51)*

Assessment	Normal Findings	Frequency
a. Vital signs		
b. Incision		
c. Ventilation		
d. Pain		
e. Urinary function		
f. Venous status		
g. Activity		
h. Gastrointestinal function		

MULTIPLE CHOICE

Directions: Select the best answer(s) for each of the following questions.

21. The patient is in the induction stage of anesthesia. Which activity will most likely be taking place? *(37)*
    1. Positioning the patient to perform the surgical procedure
    2. Decreasing the dosage(s) of anesthetic agent(s)
    3. Cleaning, shaving, and preparing the skin
    4. Establishing and verifying placement of the endotracheal tube

22. During the preoperative teaching session, a patient voices concerns about waking up during surgery. Which response should the nurse give to the patient? *(37)*
    1. "The anesthesia given during surgery will not wear off and allow you to wake up."
    2. "The anesthesiologist is able to monitor for this and will provide medications as needed."
    3. "Waking up is a risk you will face during the surgical procedure."
    4. "Emergence from anesthesia is a rare complication of surgery."

23. The patient is scheduled to undergo a urologic procedure in the surgical suite. The patient will be conscious during the procedure. What type of anesthesia will most likely be used? *(37)*
    1. Nerve block
    2. Epidural anesthesia
    3. Spinal anesthesia
    4. Local anesthesia

24. The patient is scheduled to undergo the removal of a benign cyst from his hand in the health care provider's office. The nurse is aware that the health care provider will most likely use which type of anesthesia? *(38)*
    1. Regional anesthesia
    2. Local anesthesia
    3. Conscious sedation
    4. Intrathecal anesthesia

25. The nurse is preparing to assist the health care provider who is performing a procedure using conscious sedation. Which nursing action is the most important during the procedure? *(38)*
    1. Monitoring intake and output
    2. Administering the medication
    3. Reassuring the patient
    4. Assessment of vital signs

26. The nurse is preparing an in-service for nursing staff on conscious sedation. What should be emphasized in the presentation? *(39)*
    1. The recovery from the procedure is often risky.
    2. The patient should not be prematurely extubated.
    3. Resuscitation equipment should be readily available.
    4. Nurses should not administer central nervous system depressants.

27. When developing the plan of care for an Arab American undergoing surgery, what cultural consideration may be of concern? *(19)*
    1. Stoicism during pain and discomfort
    2. Expected submissive role of women
    3. Need for a written consent for surgery
    4. Avoidance of sustained eye contact

28. Preoperative teaching is ideally provided: *(22)*
    1. 1 to 2 days before surgery.
    2. the morning of surgery.
    3. at least 2 weeks preoperatively.
    4. when the nurse has extra time.

29. Before surgery of the bowel, neomycin, sulfonamides, or erythromycin may be given to: *(24)*
    1. decrease likelihood of bowel perforation.
    2. prevent urinary tract infections.
    3. detoxify the gastrointestinal tract.
    4. reduce the risk of pneumonia.

30. The nurse is providing care for a patient in the PACU who had an unexpected surgical procedure performed. The patient has been on antihypertensive medications for a long time. What side effects related to use of antihypertensive medications should the nurse monitor for? (Select all that apply.) *(36)*
    1. Tachycardia
    2. Hypotension
    3. Bradycardia
    4. Impaired circulation
    5. Diaphoresis

31. The patient is instructed to discontinue taking nonsteroidal antiinflammatory drugs (NSAIDs) for several days before surgery. What is the best explanation for the need to hold this medication? *(36)*
    1. "NSAIDs increase susceptibility to postoperative bleeding."
    2. "NSAIDs impair healing during the postoperative period."
    3. "NSAIDs interact with the medications used for anesthesia."
    4. "NSAIDs are associated with an increase in postoperative infections."

32. A mastectomy is scheduled for an 81-year-old patient. What is the highest priority during the immediate postoperative recovery period? *(44)*
    1. Assessing for confusion
    2. Airway management
    3. Pain management
    4. Monitoring bleeding

33. The patient is being prepared to go to the operating room. With proper instructions, which task(s) can be delegated to the UAP? (Select all that apply.) *(18)*
    1. Compare current vital signs to baseline measurements.
    2. Assist the patient to remove personal clothing and don a hospital gown.
    3. Check the IV pump rate and the IV insertion site.
    4. Assist the patient to move from the bed to the stretcher.
    5. Ensure that the preoperative checklist is complete.
    6. Apply antiembolic stockings.

34. The nurse is performing preoperative teaching for a patient who must undergo a breast biopsy. The patient begins to cry softly and says, "I can't believe this is happening to me." What response should the nurse use first? *(20)*
    1. "Do you need more information about the procedure?"
    2. "The biopsy is a minor procedure, there are very few risks."
    3. "Don't cry, everything will be okay; we'll take care of you."
    4. "You seem scared; tell me what you are thinking about."

35. Which patient is most likely to have problems related to medications that are given in the perioperative setting? *(19)*
    1. A 23-year-old woman who believes in alternative and complementary medicines
    2. A 73-year-old woman who takes multiple medications for several chronic conditions
    3. A 56-year-old man who has recently started an oral antidiabetic medication
    4. A 7-year-old child who occasionally uses a rescue inhaler for asthma

36. The patient tells the nurse that he has been smoking for years and is likely to continue to smoke before and after his surgery. Which piece of equipment will the nurse emphasize during the preoperative teaching? *(26)*
    1. Normal range for pulse oximeter
    2. Use of incentive spirometer
    3. Use of patient-controlled analgesia pump
    4. Operation of the call bell

37. The nurse is evaluating the patient's understanding of the preoperative teaching. Which question should the nurse ask? *(52)*
    1. Do you have any questions about postoperative care?
    2. Would you like written information about the care plan?
    3. Did you understand everything I told you about the care?
    4. What questions do you have about the postoperative care?

38. The health care provider is preparing to explain a procedure to the patient and obtain informed consent. Which information is the most vital to relate to the provider before he/she enters the patient's room? *(23)*
    1. Patient has been talking about refusing the surgery.
    2. Patient had a hypoglycemic episode 3 hours ago.
    3. Patient's laboratory reports are not available yet.
    4. Patient received morphine and a sedative 1 hour ago.

39. The patient is on NPO status starting at midnight the night before surgery. Which task can be delegated to the UAP? *(23)*
    1. Give the patient small sips of water if he reports thirst.
    2. Assist with oral care, but instruct the patient not to swallow fluids.
    3. Obtain small hard candy for the patient to suck on.
    4. Check the patient's intravenous fluids every 2 hours.

40. Which patient would not be instructed to cough after surgery? *(28)*
    1. The patient who had abdominal surgery
    2. The patient who had pneumonia before surgery
    3. The patient who had intracranial surgery
    4. The patient who had thoracic surgery

41. The patient had surgery at 10:00 AM. At 6:00 PM the nurse notes that the patient has not voided since returning from surgery. What should the nurse do first? *(31)*
    1. Help the patient to the toilet and open the faucet so that water runs.
    2. Palpate the symphysis pubis to determine if the bladder is distended.
    3. Call the health care provider and obtain an order for catheterization.
    4. Help the patient to get up and ambulate to stimulate urination.

42. The patient is undergoing spinal anesthesia and the patient's position has to be slightly adjusted during the procedure. Which occurrence is cause for greatest concern? *(37)*
    1. Slight decrease in blood pressure
    2. Loss of sensation in both feet
    3. Slowing of respiratory rate
    4. Inability to freely move the legs

43. A patient who had surgery on the left hip tells the nurse, "You might think I am crazy, but my right arm kind of hurts since I had my surgery." What should the nurse do first? *(45)*
    1. Check the operating records for the position the patient was in during the operation.
    2. Call the health care provider and inform him/her of the new onset arm pain.
    3. Assess the arm for pulse, sensation, movement, pain, and temperature of skin.
    4. Give the patient a mild PRN pain medication and elevate the arm on a pillow.

44. Which instruction is the nurse most likely to give to the patient before administering the preoperative medication? *(34)*
    1. "Please go to the bathroom and void."
    2. "Let me mark the operative site."
    3. "I am going to take your vital signs."
    4. "Please sign the consent form."

45. The patient will soon be transferred from the PACU to the nursing unit. Which task(s) can be delegated to the UAP? (Select all that apply.) *(18)*
    1. Place the bed in a high position with side rails in appropriate position.
    2. Obtain a clean gown and extra pillows for positioning.
    3. Set up suction equipment and test function.
    4. Get stethoscope, thermometer, and sphygmomanometer.
    5. Check the function of the IV pump.
    6. Place bed pads to protect linens from drainage.

46. The anesthesia provider has written the order to transfer the patient from PACU to the nursing unit. Which assessment finding would delay the transfer? *(42, 43, 44)*
    1. Patient is awake, but nausea and some vomiting continue.
    2. Patient is breathing normally, but reports a sore throat and cough.
    3. Patient is crying and reports pain related to the surgical incision.
    4. Patient has a decreased blood pressure and pulse is increasing.

47. The patient had surgery 10 hours ago. The UAP tells the nurse that the blood pressure (BP) is 96/60 mm Hg and the patient says, "My blood pressure is usually 120/78." What should the nurse do first? *(45)*
    1. Check the patient for signs and symptoms of hypovolemic shock.
    2. Tell the UAP to go back and repeat the BP and report back.
    3. Tell the UAP to take and report BP and pulse every 5 minutes for 15 minutes.
    4. Call the health care provider and report the low reading of 96/60.

48. Which task is the responsibility of the scrub nurse? *(43)*
    1. Sends for the patient at the proper time
    2. Checks medical record for completeness
    3. Performs and confirms patient assessment
    4. Assists with surgical draping of patient

49. The nurse is preparing to discharge a patient from an ambulatory surgery setting. How does the nurse determine when the patient is ready to be discharged? *(54)*
    1. Patient states he is ready to drive himself home.
    2. Patient is groggy, but readily arouses to normal stimuli.
    3. Patient reports that pain is controlled and nausea has ceased.
    4. Family is available and willing to take responsibility.

50. The nurse is caring for a postoperative patient who has preexisting type 2 diabetes. Which assessment is most relevant to a complication associated with diabetes? *(18)*
    1. Impaired communication
    2. Bloody emesis
    3. Poor wound healing
    4. Hypoventilation

CRITICAL THINKING ACTIVITIES

Activity 1

A 35-year-old woman reports to the health care provider's office with complaints of itching; hives on her arms, neck, and chest; and sore throat. She further reports that these symptoms occur when she is at work. Further assessment reveals she works in a local nursing home in the housekeeping department. Her health history is uneventful. She is diagnosed with a latex allergy.

51. Discuss latex allergies. Include types, influencing factors, risk factors, and methods of prevention. *(24)*

_____

_____

_____

_____

_____

_____

_____

Activity 2

The health care provider informs the nurse that the patient has an unexpected problem that requires urgent surgery, which is likely to occur within the next several days.

52. Describe how the nurse can use the ABCDEF mnemonic device to ascertain serious illness or trauma in the preoperative patient. *(18)*

_____

_____

_____

_____

_____

_____

_____

Activity 3

53. Discuss four or five considerations for older adults who require surgery. *(17)*

_____

_____

_____

_____

_____

Care of the Patient with an Integumentary Disorder

Answer Key: Textbook page references are provided as a guide for answering these questions. A complete Answer Key is provided in your Additional Learning Resources on Evolve.

MATCHING

Primary Skin Lesions

Directions: Match the type of lesion on the left to the example and description on the right, and in the blank space provided indicate the letter of the correct description and example. (60-65)

Type of Lesion		Description and Example
_____	1. macule	a. Elevated irregularly shaped area of cutaneous edema; solid, transient; variable diameter (e.g., insect bite)
_____	2. papule	b. Flat, nonpalpable, irregularly shaped macule; >1 cm in diameter (e.g., port-wine stains)
_____	3. patch	c. Elevated and solid lesion; deeper in dermis; >2 cm in diameter (e.g., neoplasm)
_____	4. plaque	
_____	5. wheal	d. Elevated, circumscribed, superficial, not into dermis; filled with serous fluid; <1 cm in diameter (e.g., chickenpox)
_____	6. nodule	e. Elevated, firm, and rough lesion with flat top surface; >1 cm in diameter (e.g., psoriasis)
_____	7. tumor	
_____	8. vesicle	f. Elevated, circumscribed, encapsulated lesion; filled with liquid or semisolid material (e.g., sebaceous cyst)
_____	9. bulla	g. Dried serum, blood, or purulent exudate; slightly elevated; brown, red, black, or tan (e.g., eczema)
_____	10. pustule	
_____	11. cyst	h. Elevated, firm, circumscribed area; <1 cm in diameter [e.g., wart (verruca)]
_____	12. lichenification	i. Elevated, firm, circumscribed lesion; deeper in dermis than a papule; 1-2 cm in diameter (e.g., lipomas)
_____	13. scale	
_____	14. keloid	j. Flat, circumscribed area with a change in color; < 1 cm in diameter (e.g., freckles)
_____	15. scar	k. Irregularly shaped, progressively enlarging scar; excessive collagen (e.g., keloid formation after surgery)
_____	16. excoriation	
_____	17. fissure	l. Linear crack or break from the epidermis to the dermis; may be moist or dry (e.g., athlete's foot)
_____	18. erosion	m. Elevated, superficial lesion; similar to a vesicle but filled with purulent fluid (e.g., acne)
_____	19. ulcer	
_____	20. crust	n. Vesicle >1 cm in diameter (e.g.. blister)
_____	21. atrophy	

(Continued next page)

(Continued)

    o. Heaped-up keratinized cells; flaky skin; irregular; thick or thin; dry or oily (e.g., flaking of skin)

    p. Partial loss of the epidermis; depressed, moist, glistening; follows rupture of a vesicle (e.g., variola after rupture)

    q. Loss of epidermis and dermis; concave; varies in size (e.g., pressure sore)

    r. Thin to thick fibrous tissue that replaces normal skin after injury to the dermis (e.g., healed surgical incision)

    s. Loss of the epidermis; linear, hollowed-out, crusted area (e.g., abrasion)

    t. Rough, thickened epidermis secondary to persistent rubbing, itching (e.g., chronic dermatitis)

    u. Thinning of skin surface and loss of skin markings; skin translucent and paperlike (e.g., aged skin)

SHORT ANSWER

Directions: Using your own words, answer each question in the space provided.

22. What are the functions of the skin? *(57, 58)*

_____

_____

_____

_____

_____

23. When performing an assessment of an integumentary problem, what should be included using "PQRST"? *(66)*

_____

_____

_____

_____

24. When performing an assessment of a mole, what characteristics should be included using "ABCDE" for assessment of skin lesions? *(66)*

_____

_____

_____

_____

FIGURE LABELING

Rule of Nines

25. Directions: Label the body according to the rule of nines. *(98)*

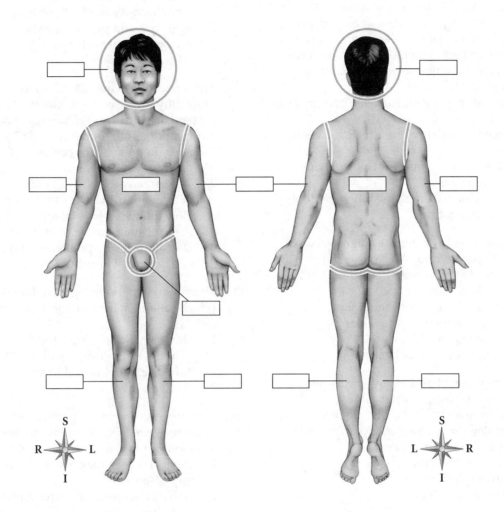

26. Calculate the percentage of burns for each of the situations listed below using the rule of nines. *(97, 98)*

    a. A 19-year-old was burned while playing with fireworks. He has burns on both of his arms (anterior and posterior) and his anterior chest. _____%

    b. A 70-year-old man was burned when he backed up into an open-flame heater. He has burns on the posterior of his body from his ankles to his neck. He also has burns on the anterior portion of his legs. _____%

    c. The patient, who has diabetes mellitus, stepped into a hot shower and has burns on his back and buttocks. _____%

MULTIPLE CHOICE

Directions: Select the best answer(s) for each of the following questions

27. The nurse hears in report that a young female patient is very upset because of alopecia; she cannot focus on the overall cancer treatment plan. In addition to therapeutic communication, which nursing intervention could the nurse use? *(88)*
    1. Suggest therapeutic baths using colloid solution.
    2. Teach the patient about use of scarves or wigs.
    3. Suggest shaving, tweezing, or rubbing with pumice.
    4. Advise the patient to use lotion immediately after bathing.

28. The health care provider has diagnosed a patient with paronychia. Which assessment is the nurse most likely to perform before administering the ordered therapy? *(96)*
    1. History of allergies to antibiotics
    2. Rating of pain on a pain scale
    3. Baseline range of motion
    4. Feelings about body image

29. A patient reports hair loss (hypotrichosis). Which assessment is the nurse mostly likely to conduct to assist the health care provider in determining the etiology of hypotrichosis? *(96)*
    1. Type of hair-care products
    2. Use of herbal supplements
    3. Smoking history
    4. Dietary assessment

30. A patient is admitted for pain and tenderness in his lower right leg. The nurse's assessment reveals that the extremity is warm, swollen, and has a slightly pitted appearance. Which measure would the nurse use to relieve the discomfort? *(76)*
    1. Assist the patient to ambulate as much as possible.
    2. Administer cool compresses or a covered icebag.
    3. Elevate the leg with pillows to reduce edema.
    4. Assist with a therapeutic bath and gently pat skin to dry.

31. When assisting a mother to plan meals for a child recently diagnosed with eczema, the nurse should advise her that common allergies for a patient with this diagnosis may include: *(83)*
    1. strawberries and cured meats.
    2. eggs, rye, and preservatives.
    3. orange juice, wheat, and eggs.
    4. wheat, sugar, and bananas

32. The nurse knows that the health care provider frequently prescribes isotretinoin (Accutane) for patients with acne. Which question is the most important to routinely ask? *(70)*
    1. Are you pregnant or contemplating a pregnancy in the near future?
    2. Do you have a history of kidney problems or frequent urinary tract infections?
    3. How often do you sunbathe? Are you willing to abstain during treatment?
    4. Do you have any problems with your liver or a history of hepatitis?

33. The nurse is interviewing an older adult. Which statement is cause for the greatest concern? *(93)*
    1. "My toenails are tough and thick."
    2. "This black mole on my neck is itching."
    3. "My hair thinning and I have a bald spot."
    4. "I have a lot of 'age spots' on my hands."

34. The nurse notes that the patient has clubbing of the fingertips. Based on this finding, which question would the nurse ask? *(60)*
    1. Have you been diagnosed with a respiratory disorder?
    2. Do you take medication for high blood pressure?
    3. Do you have a family history of diabetes mellitus?
    4. Are you taking medication for osteoporosis?

35. To assess the temperature and texture of the patient's skin, which technique would the nurse use? *(60)*
    1. Use the fingertips and gently palpate the affected area.
    2. Use the palms of the hands and compare opposite body areas.
    3. Use a cotton-tipped applicator and apply gentle pressure.
    4. Use a gloved finger to touch skin and ask about sensations.

36. The school nurse is assessing a 15-year-old girl and notices multiple linear superficial cuts over the girl's anterior forearms. What should the nurse do first? *(66)*
    1. Call child protective services to report possible abuse.
    2. Notify the girl's parents about the finding.
    3. Ask the girl directly what happened to her arms.
    4. Initiate protective measures to prevent self-harm.

37. The nurse is assessing a patient who was recently transferred from home to a skilled nursing facility. The nurse sees a pressure ulcer with full-thickness tissue loss, which is covered by a thick, black layer of eschar. What should the nurse do first? *(67)*
    1. Gently remove the eschar and check for tunneling and depth.
    2. Document the size and location of this stage IV ulcer.
    3. Contact the wound care specialist for wound management.
    4. Leave eschar intact; collaborate with RN to develop care plan.

38. The home health aide phones the nurse and says, "I helped the patient bathe. I wore gloves during the bath, but then afterwards he said that he was just diagnosed with herpes zoster." Which question would the nurse ask first? *(73)*
    1. "Are you having a painful burning rash with itching?"
    2. "Do you have fluid-filled vesicles on your back or trunk?"
    3. "Have you received two doses of varicella vaccine?"
    4. "How long were you in contact with the patient?"

39. The nurse hears during shift report that the patient was admitted for penicillin-induced dermatitis medicamentosa. Which question is the most important to ask? *(81)*
    1. Was the affected area immediately washed and rinsed?
    2. Has the patient been medicated for pain and itching?
    3. Has the patient had any respiratory distress?
    4. Does the patient have any fever or other signs of infection?

40. The nurse would be prepared to administer epinephrine as needed for which patient? *(82)*
    1. Has burning sensation and a dry crusty lesion on the lip
    2. Has a single pink, scaly patch that resembles a large ringworm
    3. Has skin maceration, fissures, and vesicles around the toes
    4. Has raised red wheals and hives and an expiratory wheeze

CRITICAL THINKING ACTIVITIES

Activity 1

41. Discuss the nursing care of a patient who has sustained a major burn through the emergent phase, acute phase, and rehabilitation phase. *(99, 100, 104)*

    a. Emergent phase _____

    _____

    _____

b. Acute phase _____

_____

_____

c. Rehabilitation phase _____

_____

_____

Activity 2

42. a. The nurse is assessing the skin of several patients. What are the physiologic factors that influence skin color? *(59, 60)*

_____

_____

_____

_____

b. Based on the patient's low hemoglobin and hematocrit, the nurse would assess for pallor. The patient is a very dark-skinned individual. How would the nurse assess this patient for pallor? *(66)*

_____

_____

_____

_____

c. The darker-skinned patient reports an itching sensation, but the nurse cannot detect a rash with visual inspection. What technique can the nurse use? *(66)*

_____

_____

_____

_____

Care of the Patient with a Musculoskeletal Disorder

Answer Key: Textbook page references are provided as a guide for answering these questions. A complete Answer Key is provided in your Additional Learning Resources on Evolve.

FIGURE LABELING

1. Directions: Label the figure of the anterior view of skeleton below with the correct names of the bones of the body. *(112)*

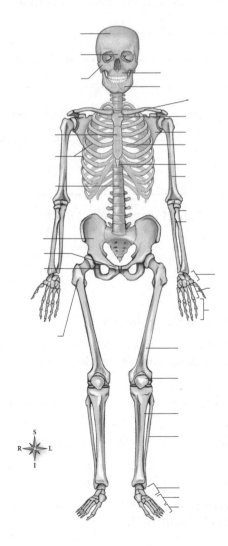

SHORT ANSWER

Directions: Using your own words, answer each question in the space provided.

2. List five functions of the skeletal system. *(110, 111)*

   a. _____

   b. _____

   c. _____

   d. _____

   e. _____

3. List three functions that muscles perform when they contract. *(111, 112)*

   a. _____

   b. _____

   c. _____

4. Discuss neurovascular assessment and include the seven Ps of orthopedic assessment. *(146)*

   _____

   _____

   _____

   _____

   _____

   _____

   _____

5. What does "RICE" mean in relation to the treatment for sprains? *(162)* _____

   _____

TRUE OR FALSE

Directions: Write T for true or F for false in the blanks provided.

___T___ 6. Following hip surgery, the nurse uses a wedge-shaped foam bolster or pillow for 7-10 days to ensure postoperative maintenance of leg adduction and to prevent dislocation of the prosthesis. *(142)*

___F___ 7. A common posture deformity is kyphosis, which is a lateral (or S) curvature of the spine. *(171)*

___T___ 8. Buck's traction is used as a temporary measure to provide support and comfort to a fractured extremity while waiting for more definitive treatment. *(141)*

___T___ 9. Approximately 50% of patients with fibromyalgia report the condition impairs their ability to successfully complete activities of daily living. *(135)*

___F___ 10. An erythrocyte sedimentation rate (ESR) is the most objective laboratory test for determining the severity of rheumatoid arthritis. *(118)*

MULTIPLE CHOICE

Directions: Select the best answer(s) for each of the following questions.

11. A patient is prescribed colchicine to treat gout. For which potential side effects associated with the medication should the nurse be assessing? *(129)*
    1. Diarrhea, nausea, and vomiting
    2. Seizures and dysrhythmias
    3. Fluid retention and sodium retention
    4. Hypercalcemia and orthostatic hypotension

12. When assisting in planning meals for a 59-year-old woman who is concerned about her risk of osteoporosis, which food should the nurse recommend as a good source of <u>calcium</u>? (Select all that apply.) *(132)*
    1. Milk
    2. Spinach
    3. Potatoes
    4. Sardines
    5. Organ meats

13. The nurse is interviewing a young woman who injured her ankle while playing soccer. With regards to the diagnostic testing that is mostly likely to be ordered, which question is the most important to ask? *(115)*
    1. Do you have allergies to seafood or iodine?
    2. Is there any chance you could be pregnant?
    3. Are you currently taking any medications?
    4. Do you have a history of radiation exposure?

14. The nurse is assessing a patient who had a myelogram 3 hours ago. Which patient comment causes the greatest concern? *(115)*
    1. "My head hurts. Could I get an aspirin or a Tylenol tablet?"
    2. "I am thirsty. Would if be okay if I drank a soda or some juice?"
    3. "My foot feels numb and I can't move my toes very well."
    4. "I am not used to lying in bed all day long; I'd like to walk around."

15. The nurse hears in report that the patient has a medical diagnosis of ankylosing spondylitis (AKS). What will the nurse include in the focused assessment for this patient? *(125)*
    1. The 7 Ps of orthopedic assessment
    2. Assessment of back pain and vision
    3. Frequent mental status checks
    4. Urinary retention and back stiffness

16. The patient says to the nurse, "I have excruciating pain in my big toe at night." Which assessment question is the nurse most likely to ask? *(129)*
    1. Have you noticed a change in your bowel movements?
    2. How much exercise would you normally get in a week?
    3. Do you eat organ meats, yeast, herring, or mackerel?
    4. Do you notice jaw tension, excessive fatigue, or anxiety?

17. The patient is admitted for acute osteomyelitis of the left lower extremity. Which instruction should the nurse give to the UAP? *(133)*
    1. Use drainage and secretion precautions when caring for the patient.
    2. Assist the patient to ambulate in the hall every 2-3 hours.
    3. Anticipate that movement is more difficult in the morning.
    4. Refresh the patient's ice pack every 2 hours or as needed.

18. The nurse is caring for a patient who had unicompartmental knee surgery. Which interventions will the nurse use in the postoperative period? (Select all that apply.) *(137)*
    1. Encourage deep-breathing and coughing every 2 hours.
    2. Begin with a clear liquid diet and advance to regular as tolerated.
    3. Inspect the skin at the edge of the cast for erythema.
    4. Assess the patient's ability to use an assistive device such as a walker.
    5. Monitor IV fluids and effectiveness of antibiotics.
    6. Administer intraarticular injections of corticosteroids.

19. The nurse is assessing a patient following a hip arthroplasty and returned from surgery early in the shift. The patient is now restless and anxious. What is the nurse's first action? *(149, 150)*
    1. Decrease anxiety by reassuring the patient that everything is going as expected.
    2. Initiate vital signs q 15 minutes, compare to baseline and monitor trends.
    3. Look at the urinary output and compare the total to baseline.
    4. Call the patient's family and invite them to spend time at the bedside.

20. A fiberglass cast has been applied to the fore-arm of a 6-year-old child to treat and stabilize a greenstick fracture. Which teaching point is the most important to emphasize with the child? *(150)*
    1. Instructing the child to keep the cast dry
    2. Teaching the child to report pain to the parents
    3. Showing the child how to test capillary refill
    4. Reminding the child to wiggle the fingers

21. The nurse is supervising a nursing student in the care of a patient who had internal fixation for a hip fracture. The nurse would intervene if the student performed which action? *(142)*
    1. Assessed the amount of drainage in the Jackson-Pratt drain
    2. Encouraged coughing and the use of the incentive spirometer
    3. Removed the antiembolism stocking to assess the skin
    4. Placed the patient in high Fowler's position prior to eating

22. The nurse is providing care for a patient who has just had a hip replacement. Which comment from the patient indicates the need for further education? *(137)*
    1. "I need to be on bedrest for the first 72 hours."
    2. "I need to obtain a seat riser for my toilet at home."
    3. "I should never sit with my legs crossed."
    4. "I'll have limitations in hip position for 2-3 months."

23. A nurse is checking on an elderly neighbor who just fell down. The man cheerfully tells the nurse, "I just tripped on the carpet and took a spill. No harm done!" Based on mechanism of injury, which assessment is the nurse most likely to perform if the neighbor will allow it? *(145)*
    1. Head-to-toe to detect occult injury
    2. Palpation and range of motion for wrist injury
    3. Mental status examination for head injury
    4. Environmental assessment for other hazards

24. The patient was in a car accident and reports pain over the pelvic region with difficulty raising legs in a supine position. The nurse notes ecchymosis over the pelvic region. Which laboratory test is the primary concern in the immediate phase of care? *(149)*
    1. Hemoglobin and hematocrit
    2. Blood type and Rh
    3. Urinalysis
    4. Stool for occult blood

25. The patient with a cast on the lower extremity reports pain at 7/10. What should the nurse do first? *(141)*
    1. Reposition the leg so that elevation is maintained.
    2. Administer pain medication as ordered.
    3. Report potential compartment syndrome to RN.
    4. Perform the 7 Ps of orthopedic assessment.

26. The nurse hears in report that the patient has Volkmann's contracture of the dominant upper extremity. Which intervention would the nurse plan to use? *(150)*
    1. Frequent assessment using the 7 Ps of orthopedic assessment
    2. Assess the patient's abilities to perform activities of daily living
    3. Teach the patient to report pain, loss of sensation, or swelling
    4. Instruct the UAP on how to maintain proper position and alignment

27. The nurse is caring for a patient with a long bone fracture. The laboratory reports the following arterial blood gas results. What should the nurse do first? *(152)*

pH	7.4
$Paco_2$	40 mm Hg
Pao_2	95 mm Hg
HCO_3	26 mEq/L
Sao_2	98%

   1. Assess the patient for signs of fat embolism and respiratory distress.
   2. Report these normal results to the health care provider.
   3. Place the patient in high Fowler's position to ease respirations.
   4. Check the vital signs and continue to monitor the patient.

28. A computer data entry clerk reports paresthesia in the thumb, index finger, and middle finger and pain that increases during the night. The clerk has an appointment with a health care provider next week. In the meantime, what self-care measure would the nurse advise? *(165, 166)*
   1. Use warm packs and sleep with hands on a pillow.
   2. Frequently change position and stretch hands while working.
   3. Use a mild analgesic such as ibuprofen or aspirin.
   4. Wrap the wrist snugly with an elastic bandage.

29. The patient who had a laminectomy reports abdominal discomfort with a gaseous, bloated feeling and mild nausea. What should the nurse do first? *(167)*
   1. Offer clear liquids
   2. Encourage ambulation
   3. Listen for bowel sounds
   4. Administer an antiemetic

30. The patient reports long bone pain that increases with weight-bearing. The health care provider tells the nurse that the patient has an elevated serum alkaline phosphatase. The nurse prepares to give emotional support because the health care provider must tell the patient that additional diagnostic testing is need to rule out: *(168)*
   1. phantom limb pain.
   2. compartment syndrome.
   3. fibromyalgia.
   4. osteogenic sarcoma.

CRITICAL THINKING ACTIVITIES

Activity 1

31. Discuss factors that contribute to osteoporosis and the nurse's role in helping patients prevent bone loss and fractures. *(130)*

_____

_____

_____

_____

_____

_____

Activity 2

32. A 32-year-old woman has been told that she might have fibromyalgia syndrome; however, the health care provider tells her that this is just a possibility and that additional diagnostic testing would be needed. The patient is angry at first and then she begins to cry and confides in the nurse, "I am just so frustrated with these doctors and I just want to be able to live a normal life." Discuss fibromyalgia syndrome from the patient's point of view. *(132-135)*

_____

_____

_____

_____

_____

Activity 3

33. The home health nurse is visiting a thin elderly woman who lives alone. The three-story house is a little cluttered with old belongings. Her bedroom and bathroom are on the second floor. The rugs are worn and the hallways are poorly lit. The woman cheerfully reports that she has a cane, a walker, and eyeglasses, but frequently misplaces "all of the 'old person' stuff." The woman has a small friendly dog; he jumps at her legs and she frequently bends down to pet him. Discuss the potential for hip fracture for this woman. *(140)*

_____

_____

_____

_____

_____

Activity 4

34. A patient diagnosed with rheumatoid arthritis requests additional information. She states that she has heard of two types of arthritis. She asks about the differences between rheumatoid arthritis and osteoarthritis. Compare and contrast rheumatoid arthritis and osteoarthritis. Include cause, clinical manifestations, treatment options, and prognosis. *(119-128)*

_____

_____

_____

_____

_____

_____

Care of the Patient with a Gastrointestinal Disorder

Answer Key: Textbook page references are provided as a guide for answering these questions. A complete Answer Key is provided in your Additional Learning Resources on Evolve.

FIGURE LABELING

1. Directions: Label the digestive organs. *(177)*

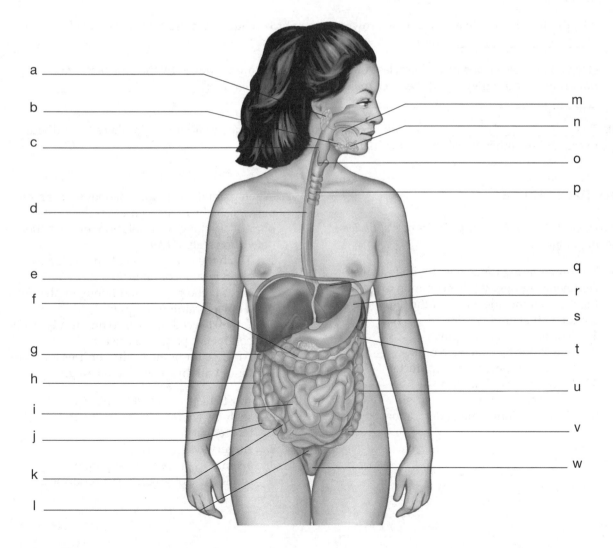

a _____

b _____

c _____

d _____

e _____

f _____

g _____

h _____

i _____

j _____

k _____

l _____

m _____

n _____

o _____

p _____

q _____

r _____

s _____

t _____

u _____

v _____

w _____

FILL-IN-THE-BLANK SENTENCES

Directions: Complete each sentence by filling in the blank with the correct word or phrase.

2. _____ is the coordinated, rhythmic, sequential contraction of smooth muscle that pushes food through the digestive tract, as well as bile through the bile duct. *(176)*

3. Lysozyme is a salivary enzyme that destroys bacteria and thus protects the mucous membrane from _____ and the teeth from _____. *(178)*

4. The cardiac sphincter contracts and prevents _____, which can be irritating to the esophagus. *(178)*

5. Pancreatic juices are essential in breaking down _____ into their amino acid components, in reducing dietary _____ to glycerol and fatty acids, and in converting starch to _____. *(179)*

6. The large intestine has four major functions: (1) absorption of _____, (2) manufacture of certain vitamins (such as vitamin K and B$_7$), (3) formation of _____, and (4) _____ of feces. *(179)*

7. The bacteria in the large intestine are also responsible for the synthesis of vitamin K, which is needed for normal _____. *(180)*

8. Bile, produced in the liver, is a yellow-brown or green-brown liquid necessary for the emulsification of _____. *(180)*

9. (Trypsin), lipase (steapsin), and amylase (amylopsin), which are produced by the pancreas, are important because they digest the three major components of chyme: _____, _____, and _____. *(191)*

10. The _____, a portion of the brain, contains one center that stimulates the individual to eat, and the other signals the individual to stop eating. *(181)*

MULTIPLE CHOICE

Directions: Select the best answer(s) for each of the following questions.

11. The nurse caring for a patient with fecal incontinence recognizes that common causes of the disorder include which of the following? (Select all that apply.) *(228)*
    1. Normal changes of aging
    2. Injury during anal intercourse
    3. Surgical trauma to anal sphincter
    4. Injury during childbirth
    5. Spinal cord lesions
    6. Voluntary inhibition of defecation

12. When planning care for a patient with a motor paralysis, which intervention is the most important as a long-term solution for the patient's defecation status? *(228)*
    1. Teach the family and patient the log roll to clean fecal incontinence.
    2. Include the patient and family in planning a bowel training program.
    3. Contact social services to find funds for incontinence pads and briefs.
    4. Arrange for home health services for assistance with hygiene and toileting.

13. The most effective bowel training programs will include: *(228)*
    1. biofeedback.
    2. surgery.
    3. enemas to prevent constipation.
    4. routine use of glycerin suppositories.

14. The patient is practicing a bowel training program. Which food will the nurse encourage the patient to eat? *(228)*
    1. Lean chicken meat
    2. Low-fat milk
    3. Whole-grain cereal
    4. Red meat

15. A patient is being treated with sucralfate (Carafate) for gastroesophageal reflux disease (GERD). Which teaching point would the nurse emphasize? *(196)*
    1. Oral anticoagulants, theophylline, and propranolol may require dosage reductions.
    2. Coating action may interfere with the absorption of other drugs—separate by 2 hours.
    3. Contraindicated during pregnancy; women of childbearing age must use reliable contraception.
    4. Avoid driving or other hazardous activities until accustomed to sedating effects.

16. A patient had a partial gastrectomy. Because this surgery creates an increased risk for pernicious anemia, which teaching point is important to emphasize? *(202)*
    1. Blood serum vitamin B_{12} level should be measured every 1 to 2 years.
    2. Hemoglobin and hematocrit should be measured every 1 to 2 months.
    3. Injections of iron dextran (DexFerrum) are given because of intestinal ulceration.
    4. Increase fresh fruits and vegetables, and decrease intake of fat and red meat.

17. The risk of cancer of the stomach is associated with which factors? (Select all that apply.) *(199)*
    1. Hyperkalemia
    2. Hypochlorhydria
    3. Chronic atrophic gastritis
    4. Diet high in smoked and preserved foods
    5. Gastric ulcers
    6. Diet high in fresh fruits and whole grains

18. When caring for a patient diagnosed with Crohn's disease, what signs and symptoms does the nurse expect to observe? (Select all that apply.) *(212)*
    1. Nausea and vomiting
    2. Diarrhea and abdominal pain
    3. Weight gain and lactose intolerance
    4. Weight loss and malnutrition
    5. Fatigue and fever

19. The nurse is providing care to a patient suspected of having acute appendicitis. Which interventions may be included in care? (Select all that apply.) *(214)*
    1. Apply heating pad to the abdomen.
    2. Maintain bedrest and nothing by mouth (NPO).
    3. Administer PRN antacids to decrease gastric acidity.
    4. Monitor vital signs including temperature.
    5. Administer antibiotics as ordered.
    6. Administer enemas until clear.

20. The patient had an esophagogastroduodenoscopy several hours ago and now reports abdominal pain and tenderness to the nurse. What should the nurse do first? *(182)*
    1. Auscultate for bowel sounds
    2. Administer pain medication
    3. Assess the abdominal pain
    4. Check for melena

21. The patient had capsule endoscopy. Which discharge instruction should the nurse give to the patient? *(182)*
    1. Return in 8 hours to have the monitoring device removed.
    2. Examine stool for several days to retrieve pill camera device.
    3. Use a mild laxative to facilitate expulsion of pill camera.
    4. Small amounts of blood and mucus in the stool are expected.

22. The nurse inserts a nasosgastric tube (NG) so a patient can undergo the Bernstein test to determine the cause of esophageal pain. Which outcome is considered a positive test result? *(182, 183)*
    1. Administering nitrates relieves pain.
    2. Taking an antacid has no effect on pain.
    3. Decompressing the stomach relieves pain.
    4. Instilling hydrochloric acid causes pain.

23. The patient needs to have a series of tests for the gastrointestinal system. Which test must be scheduled last? *(184)*
    1. Barium studies
    2. Stool sample for ova and parasites
    3. Colonoscopy
    4. Flat plate of the abdomen

24. The nursing student reports seeing a pearly, bluish-white "milk-curd" on the mucous membranes of the older patient's mouth. The nurse would intervene if the student performs which action? *(185)*
    1. Checks for angular cheilitis at the corner of the mouth
    2. Removes the plaques with a soft toothbrush
    3. Observes the quantity and type of food consumed
    4. Offers the patient unsweetened yogurt

25. The nurse is talking to a neighbor who says that she has had a sore on her lip for about 3 weeks. What advice should the nurse give? *(186)*
    1. Use lipstick or lip balm that has includes a sunscreen.
    2. Advise rinsing the mouth with diluted hydrogen peroxide.
    3. Consult the health care provider because of the duration of the sore.
    4. Increase intake of fresh fruits and vegetables for vitamin content.

26. The health care provider has recommended a conservative approach to manage the patient's gastroesophageal reflux disease (GERD). What would be included in the nurse's instructions to support the provider's recommendation? *(188)*
    1. Give the patient a brochure about Nissen fundoplication.
    2. Suggest methods for elevating the head of the bed at home.
    3. Teach the signs and symptoms of Barrett's esophagus.
    4. Give the patient a reminder card for endoscopy and biopsy.

27. The nurse is caring for a patient who was admitted for peptic ulcer disease. Which diagnostic finding is greatest cause for concern? *(182)*
    1. Fecal assay antigen test is positive for *H. pylori*.
    2. Stool for occult blood is positive.
    3. White blood cell count is elevated.
    4. Pain is present during the hydrochloric acid test.

28. The patient who had surgery for a peptic ulcer several weeks ago reports experiencing an episode of diaphoresis, nausea, vomiting, epigastric pain, explosive diarrhea, and dyspepsia. Which question is most relevant to the symptoms and the surgical history? *(201)*
    1. Can you describe the pain? Where was it and how long did it last?
    2. Did you eat before the symptoms? And if so, what did you eat?
    3. Have you been taking your medications according to instructions?
    4. Did you ever experience these symptoms before the surgery?

29. The patient is admitted for hemorrhagic colitis caused by the *E. coli* pathogen. Which order would the nurse question? *(203)*
    1. Encourage oral fluids as tolerated
    2. Dextrose 5% in normal saline at 150 mL/hour
    3. Loperamide (Imodium) 2 mg after unformed stool
    4. Initiate contact isolation

30. The elderly patient has been put into contact isolation because of watery diarrhea. Laboratory results are pending, but the *C. difficile* pathogen is suspected. What instruction should the nurse give to the UAP? *(203)*
    1. Cluster care and limit the amount of time spent in the room.
    2. Use diluted bleach solution to clean the toilet bowl after each use.
    3. Wear a mask during patient care and discard upon exiting the room.
    4. Use soap and water to wash hands, rather than the antiseptic hand rub.

31. A patient who is diagnosed with celiac sprue must be taught to avoid which food? *(205)*
    1. Fish
    2. Rice
    3. Meat
    4. Wheat

32. The patient confides in the nurse that she feels angry because the health care provider has hinted that irritable bowel syndrome (IBS) might be the problem, but offers no definitive diagnosis. What is the most therapeutic response? *(207)*
    1. "IBS is hard to diagnose. It is more a process of excluding other disorders."
    2. "I'll ask the health care provider to talk to you about your concerns."
    3. "You seem really frustrated. What has the provider told you so far?"
    4. "I can get some literature about IBS; maybe additional information will help."

33. The patient is admitted for an exacerbation of ulcerative colitis and the nurse hears in report that the patient had 20 liquid stools within the past 24 hours. Which laboratory result is the most important to query? *(209)*
    1. Electrolyte levels
    2. Liver function studies
    3. Hemoglobin and hematocrit
    4. Fecal occult blood

34. The nurse enters the room of a young woman and sees that she is crying. The patient states, "The doctor told me I need surgery and an ileostomy. I'll be pooping into a bag! I'm leaving the hospital right now!" What should the nurse do first? *(210)*
    1. Obtain a Leaving Against Medical Advice form and contact the provider.
    2. Sit with the patient and help her verbalize her fears and concerns.
    3. Arrange for the patient to meet another person who has an ostomy.
    4. Contact the enterostomal therapist to talk with the patient.

35. Which medical diagnosis requires that the nurse be extra vigilant for concurrent urinary tract infections? *(212)*
    1. Crohn's disease
    2. Appendicitis
    3. Ulcerative colitis
    4. Peptic ulcer disease

36. A parent says, "I think my son has appendicitis. He won't eat and he says he has pain just to the right of his belly button." If the nurse places the child on an examination table, which position is the child most likely to assume if the mother is correct about appendicitis? *(214)*
    1. Prone with head supported by forearm
    2. Supine with arms and legs extended
    3. Sits upright, with chest extended
    4. Side-lying with knees flexed

37. The patient is admitted for acute diverticulitis. The nurse would intervene if a nursing student performed which action? *(216)*
    1. Advises to avoid heavy lifting
    2. Assists with a meal tray
    3. Assesses bowel sounds
    4. Checks the white blood cell count

38. A patient sustained blunt trauma to the abdomen. Several hours after being admitted for observation, the patient reports severe abdominal pain with exquisite tenderness to light palpation. What should the nurse do first? *(217)*
    1. Take vital signs and perform additional assessment of the abdomen.
    2. Place the patient in a semi-Fowler's position to localize purulent drainage.
    3. Call the health care provider and report possible peritonitis.
    4. Administer a PRN pain medication and reevaluate pain in 30 minutes.

39. The nurse is caring for a patient who had a right hemicolectomy for colorectal cancer. Which postoperative interventions will the nurse use in the care of this patient? (Select all that apply.) *(225)*
    1. Monitor vital signs, pain level, and return of bowel sounds.
    2. Check dressings for drainage and bleeding and change as ordered.
    3. Discontinue the Foley catheter when the patient is discharged.
    4. Encourage the patient to cough, deep-breathe, and turn.
    5. Maintain bedrest while the nasogastric tube is on suction.
    6. Keep accurate intake and output records to monitor fluid balance.

40. An obese male truck driver reports to the clinic complaining of rectal itching. After the medical examination, a diagnosis of hemorrhoids is made. What nonsurgical approaches can the nurse teach the patient to help manage the condition? *(226)*
    1. Suggest a low-fiber diet.
    2. Advise the use of a hydrocortisone cream.
    3. Increase fluid intake.
    4. Recommend rubber-band ligation.

CRITICAL THINKING ACTIVITIES

Activity 1

41. For each phase of the nursing process, indicate specifically how that phase relates to patients with esophageal disorders. *(229)*

    a. Assessment: _____

    _____

    b. Nursing diagnoses and planning: _____

    _____

    c. Implementation: _____

    _____

    d. Evaluation: _____

    _____

Activity 2

42. For each topic, list the nursing interventions appropriate for a patient who is having gastric surgery. *(202)*

    a. Preoperative

        i. Preparation: _____

        _____

        ii. Knowledge: _____

        _____

    b. Postoperative

        i. Knowledge: _____

        _____

        ii. Pain: _____

        _____

iii. Noncompliance: _____

_____

iv. Nutrition: _____

_____

Activity 3

43. The nurse is providing care to a patient suspected of having an intestinal obstruction. *(220, 221)*

a. When performing an assessment on the patient, what objective data should be included?

_____

_____

b. What diagnostic tests may be performed to confirm the presence of an intestinal obstruction?

_____

_____

c. What are the goals of treatment for an intestinal obstruction?_____

_____

_____

d. Compare and contrast mechanical and nonmechanical intestinal obstruction._____

_____

_____

Care of the Patient with a Gallbladder, Liver, Biliary Tract, or Exocrine Pancreatic Disorder

chapter

6

Answer Key: Textbook page references are provided as a guide for answering these questions. A complete Answer Key is provided in your Additional Learning Resources on Evolve.

MATCHING

Directions: Match the word or prefix on the left with the definition on the right and indicate the correct answer in the space provided.

Word or prefix

_____ 1. sphincter of Oddi *(253)*

_____ 2. T-tube *(254)*

_____ 3. cholangiography *(235)*

_____ 4. HIDA scan *(235)*

_____ 5. laparoscopic cholecystectomy *(254)*

_____ 6. cholecystectomy *(253)*

_____ 7. cholecystitis *(252)*

_____ 8. cholecystography *(234)*

_____ 9. cholecystostomy *(256)*

_____ 10. T-tube cholangiogram *(235)*

_____ 11. choledocholithiasis *(256)*

_____ 12. cholangiomas *(245)*

_____ 13. lithotripsy *(253)*

_____ 14. cholelithiasis *(252)*

Definitions

a. Biliary drainage tube
b. Hepatobiliary iminodiacetic acid scan
c. Presence of gallstones
d. Stones in common bile duct
e. Postoperative cholangiography
f. Radiographic examination of bile ducts
g. Radiographic examination of gallbladder
h. Removal of gallbladder
i. Controls the flow of pancreatic juices and bile into the duodenum
j. Laser or cautery is used to remove the gallbladder
k. Incision into the gallbladder (usually for drainage)
l. Biliary duct carcinomas
m. Inflammation of gallbladder
n. Series of shock waves through water or a cushion that breaks the stones into fragments

FILL-IN-THE-BLANK SENTENCES

15. Jaundice, the _____ of body tissues caused by abnormally high blood levels of bilirubin, is visible when the total serum bilirubin exceeds _____. *(233)*

16. Chances for developing alcohol-related cirrhosis increase for women when they ingest more than _____ alcoholic drinks per day, and for men when they drink _____ drinks per day. *(238)*

17. Cirrhosis of the liver and infection with hepatitis C or hepatitis B are factors in increased risk for primary _____ cancer. *(245)*

18. There are approximately _____ people waiting for liver transplants; currently, only approximately 6000 transplants are performed annually. *(249)*

19. More than 90% of cholecystitis cases are caused by _____. *(252)*

20. The most common lifestyle risk factor for pancreatic cancer is _____. *(259)*

MULTIPLE CHOICE

Directions: Select the best answer(s) for each of the following questions.

21. The nurse is providing teaching to a patient scheduled to undergo a needle liver biopsy. During the examination, the patient should be advised to: *(236)*
    1. deeply inhale and hold breath until told to exhale.
    2. cough forcefully as the needle is withdrawn.
    3. inhale and exhale slowly and evenly as the needle is inserted.
    4. exhale and not breathe as the needle is inserted.

22. A T-tube was inserted during a cholecystectomy. What does the nurse expect to observe when assessing the patient? *(254)*
    1. Greenish-yellow drainage from the tube
    2. Localized inflammation around the tube site
    3. Significant postoperative pain until the tube is removed
    4. Moderate amount of light-red bleeding from the tube

23. After a laparoscopic cholecystectomy, the patient reports shoulder pain. What should the nurse do? *(255)*
    1. Perform gentle range-of-motion exercises to reduce shoulder discomfort.
    2. Assist the patient to ambulate to clear the residual carbon dioxide.
    3. Explain that the pain is a side effect of anesthesia.
    4. Reassure that the pain is expected and give an analgesic as ordered.

24. When caring for a patient with acute pancreatitis, which laboratory finding is the best indicator of the disorder? *(237)*
    1. Low albumin
    2. Elevated lipase
    3. Increased blood glucose
    4. Elevated amylase

25. Which behavior places the patient at greatest risk to contract hepatitis E? *(247)*
    1. Drinking water from a questionable source
    2. Engaging in unprotected anal and vaginal sex
    3. Sharing and reusing needles for illicit drug injection
    4. Traveling to Europe, Asia, or Australia

26. The nurse is talking to a patient who had an outpatient oral cholecystogram with poor visualization of the biliary tree. What question would the nurse ask to determine if the patient was compliant with the preparation for the test? *(234)*
    1. "Did you take the laxative and the enema as directed by the health care provider?"
    2. "How many dye tablets did you take on the evening before the examination?"
    3. "When was the last time you had a meal that contained a lot of fiber?"
    4. "How much fluid did you consume on the morning of the examination?"

27. A young woman who is pregnant is having symptoms of cholecystitis and the health care provider has informed her that diagnostic testing is required. Which information brochure will the nurse prepare for this patient? *(235)*
    1. "What You Need to Know About Ultrasonography for the Gallbladder"
    2. "Frequently Asked Questions About Oral Cholecystography"
    3. "Intravenous Cholangiography: A Patient's Guide for Decision-making"
    4. "Computed Tomography of the Abdomen as a Diagnostic Tool"

28. The patient had a hepatobiliary iminodiacetic acid (HIDA) scan. What instructions should the nurse give to the UAP who is assisting the patient with hygiene? *(235)*
    1. Immediately flush all urine and stool.
    2. Wear your personal dosimeter at all times.
    3. Give care as usual; there are no special considerations.
    4. Watch for and report any bleeding at the puncture site.

29. The nurse hears in report that several patients are scheduled for diagnostic testing. The nurse must plan to take vital signs every 15 minutes (two times), then every 30 minutes (four times), and then every hour (four times) after which test? *(236)*
    1. Serum ammonia test
    2. Needle liver biopsy
    3. Oral cholecystography
    4. Radioisotope liver scan

30. The nurse is instructing the UAP about assisting several patients with morning hygiene. Which patient needs to use a soft toothbrush with very gentle brushing action? *(244)*
    1. Recently diagnosed with hepatitis A
    2. Surgery pending for cholelithiasis
    3. In later stage of cirrhosis of the liver
    4. NPO for acute pancreatitis

31. A first-semester nursing student tells the nurse that she would like to teach and coach coughing and deep-breathing for several patients. Which patient(s) would be best for the nurse to recommend to the student? (Select all that apply.) *(250, 255)*
    1. Scheduled to have a cholecystectomy in two days
    2. Looks forward to having a liver transplant from a living donor
    3. Has cirrhosis of the liver and esophageal varices
    4. Prescribed several weeks of bedrest for chronic hepatitis
    5. Is on bedrest for acute pancreatitis with severe pain

32. The patient has symptoms of hepatic encephalopathy and the health care provider wants to be called about laboratory results. Which laboratory result should the nurse seek out to validate the suspected condition? *(236)*
    1. Serum bilirubin
    2. Serum albumin
    3. Ammonia level
    4. Blood glucose

33. The health care provider orders an intramuscular immune serum globulin for a hospital employee who was exposed to hepatitis A. A dosage of 0.02 mL/kg of body weight is ordered. The employee weighs 155 lbs. How many mL should the nurse draw up? _____ *(248)*

34. A patient with acute pancreatitis is refusing to have a nasogastric tube inserted and wants to leave the hospital. What can the nurse say to help the patient to accept the therapy? *(257)*
    1. "I can give you pain medication before or after the procedure."
    2. "Let me call the health care provider so he can explain the therapy."
    3. "The tube will be inserted by our most experienced nurse, so don't worry."
    4. "The tube will decrease the nausea, vomiting, pain, and abdominal distention."

CRITICAL THINKING ACTIVITIES

Activity 1

35. A 34-year-old patient with a history of end-stage liver disease related to chronic hepatitis has been added to the waiting list to receive a liver transplant. During his preoperative education classes, he voices many questions and concerns. *(249, 250)*

   a. What are the primary risks associated with the planned transplant? _____

   _____

   b. What postoperative complications will the patient be at risk for?_____

   _____

   _____

   c. How will the risk of organ rejection be handled?_____

   _____

   _____

   _____

   d. Discuss the appropriate postoperative nursing care._____

   _____

   _____

   _____

Activity 2

36. A 49-year-old patient comes to the emergency department complaining of right upper-quadrant pain. She reports that the pain began a few hours after eating at a local fast-food restaurant. Upon assessment, the abdomen is distended. The patient also has nausea and vomiting. *(252, 253)*

   a. What does the nurse expect the patient to be diagnosed with? _____

   b. What are some other signs and symptoms that may develop? _____

   _____

   c. What diagnostic examinations may be used to help diagnose this patient? _____

   _____

   _____

   _____

Activity 3

37. a.   Based on knowledge of the etiology and clinical course of pancreatic cancer, discuss some of the psychological challenges that a patient could face. *(260)*

_____

_____

_____

_____

   b.   What can the nurse do to assist the patient with these psychological challenges? _____

_____

_____

_____

_____

Care of the Patient with a Blood or Lymphatic Disorder

Answer Key: Textbook page references are provided as a guide for answering these questions. A complete Answer Key is provided in your Additional Learning Resources on Evolve.

SHORT ANSWER

Directions: Using your own words, answer each question in the space provided.

1. What are the three main functions of blood? *(265)* _____

   _____

   _____

   _____

2. What are three functions of the lymphatic system? *(269, 270)* _____

   _____

   _____

   _____

3. What are two main functions of the lymph glands? *(270)* _____

   _____

   _____

4. What are five functions of the spleen? *(270, 271)* _____

   _____

   _____

   _____

   _____

   _____

TRUE OR FALSE

Directions: Write T for true or F for false in the blanks provided.

_____   5.   Blood is slightly acidic, with a pH range of 7.05 to 7.25. *(265)*

_____   6.   Body defense, such as the destruction of bacteria and viruses, is the primary function of the red blood cells. *(267)*

_____   7.   Using the posterior superior iliac crest for bone marrow aspiration creates the greatest risk for penetrating the underlying structures during the procedure. *(271)*

_____   8.   *Pancytopenia* means that all three major blood elements (red cells, white cells, and platelets) from the bone marrow are reduced or absent. *(277)*

_____   9.   A patient with aplastic anemia could have symptoms related to infection, decreased oxygenation of tissues, and bleeding tendencies. *(277)*

_____   10.   Hematopoietic stem cell transplant is the only available therapy with curative intent for sickle cell disease. *(282)*

TABLE ACTIVITY

11. Directions: Complete the table below with the normal values for selected blood tests. *(265)*

Blood Test	Normal Values
Red blood cells (RBCs)	Males: Females:
Hemoglobin	Males: Females:
Hematocrit	Males: Females:
Platelet count	
White blood cells (WBC) actual cell count	
Prothrombin time (PT)	
International Normalized Ratio (INR)	
Partial thromboplastin time (PTT)	

MULTIPLE CHOICE

Directions: Select the best answer(s) for each of the following questions.

12. The nurse is caring for a young patient who has had vomiting and diarrhea secondary to food poisoning, but he is usually very healthy. What would be an expected laboratory result for this patient? *(265)*
    1. Elevated hemoglobin and hematocrit
    2. Normal hemoglobin and hematocrit
    3. Low platelet count
    4. Increased prothrombin time

13. The health care provider tells the nurse that the laboratory results show that the patient has bandemia. The nurse will plan to be extra vigilant for which condition? *(267)*
    1. Deep vein thrombosis
    2. Thrombocytopenia
    3. Sepsis or septic shock
    4. Allergic response

14. Which patient is most likely to require testing for anti-D antibodies and/or an injection of RH immunoglobulin? *(269)*
    1. An Rh-positive mother who is 28 weeks gestation
    2. Any woman who has an ectopic pregnancy
    3. An Rh-negative mother who had a miscarriage
    4. An Rh-positive mother impregnated by an Rh-negative father

15. When caring for patients who are Jehovah's Witnesses, which information applies for use of blood products? *(273)*
    1. Some Jehovah's Witnesses may permit the use of certain blood volume expanders.
    2. It is not legal for this patient to refuse transfusions if the bleeding is truly life-threatening.
    3. Some Jehovah's Witnesses may consent to homologous blood transfusions.
    4. Jehovah's Witnesses believe that children are allowed to have blood in an emergency.

16. A patient with anemia has a nursing diagnosis of Activity Intolerance related to tissue hypoxia. Which task can be delegated to the UAP? *(273)*
    1. Ask the patient how far he is able to ambulate and evaluate his abilities.
    2. Apply oxygen per nasal cannula if the patient reports shortness of breath.
    3. Explain the patient's limitations to visitors and encourage short visits.
    4. Assist the patient with self-care activities, such as hygiene and toileting.

17. The nurse is caring for a trauma patient who must be observed for signs and symptoms of occult bleeding and injury. Which sign/symptom is an early manifestation of hypovolemic shock? *(274)*
    1. Orthostatic blood pressure
    2. Decreased red blood cell count
    3. Restlessness
    4. Decreased urine output

18. The patient had major abdominal surgery yesterday. He reported abdominal pain, and the nurse gave him an opioid pain medication as directed; 2 hours later, he reports that the pain is worse. What should the nurse do first? *(274)*
    1. Check the medication administration record for other pain or adjunctive medications.
    2. Explain to the patient that pain medication can only be given as ordered every 4 to 6 hours.
    3. Reassess the abdomen and ask the patient to describe the pain to the best of his ability.
    4. Call the health care provider and obtain an order for laboratory studies or x-ray studies.

19. The nurse is caring for a postoperative patient who is demonstrating early symptoms of hypovolemic shock. The nurse is awaiting a return call from the health care provider. Which task can be delegated to the UAP? *(275)*
    1. Take and report the blood pressure, pulse, and respirations every 15 minutes.
    2. Reinforce the dressings for saturation of blood or drainage.
    3. Apply oxygen and monitor the pulse oximetry readings every 5 minutes.
    4. Place the patient in a supine position and monitor respiratory effort.

20. The health care provider has recommended that the patient with sickle cell disease have a splenectomy. Which medication is likely to be discontinued for several days prior to the surgery? *(278)*
    1. Diuretic medication
    2. Vitamin B_{12}
    3. Blood thinner
    4. Blood pressure medication

21. The nurse is caring for a patient experiencing an initial sickle cell crisis. What is the primary sign/symptom that the nurse should expect during the crisis? *(281)*
    1. Jaundice
    2. Fever
    3. Fatigue
    4. Pain

22. What health promotion points should be emphasized for patients who have sickle cell disease? (Select all that apply.) *(282)*
    1. Avoid high altitudes
    2. Drink large amounts of iced fluids
    3. Stay current with vaccinations
    4. Maintain very cold room temperatures
    5. Stop smoking and alcohol consumption
    6. Maintain vigorous exercise routine

23. The patient is diagnosed with primary polycythemia. Which assessments are of particular concern? *(283)*
    1. Palpating for abdominal distention and checking bowel movements
    2. Checking for pain, warmth, swelling, redness, and pulses in arms or legs
    3. Monitoring temperature and watching for other signs of infection
    4. Frequently assessing for fatigue and activity intolerance

24. The laboratory calls to inform the nurse that the patient has a white cell count of $1000/mm^3$ with a differential neutrophil count of less than $200/mm^3$. Which action is the most important for the nurse to initiate while waiting for the health care provider to respond to the phone message? *(285)*
    1. Review current medication list.
    2. Start protective isolation precautions.
    3. Check for signs/symptoms of infection.
    4. Teach the importance of hand hygiene.

25. A 6-year-old child is hospitalized for treatment of acute lymphocytic leukemia. Which activity would the nurse suggest to the child and parents? *(288)*
    1. Drawing pictures that accompany storytelling
    2. Playing with and petting the pet therapy dog
    3. Walking in the garden courtyard
    4. Attending a party in the pediatric play area

26. The nurse is examining the patient and notices several areas of ecchymoses and petechiae. Which question(s) will the nurse ask to follow up on this observation? (Select all that apply.) *(289, 290)*
    1. What do you think is causing these bruises?
    2. Do you notice any bleeding when you brush your teeth?
    3. Have you had frequent nosebleeds?
    4. Are your stools a black or very dark red color?
    5. Are you using a hydrocortisone cream on these areas?
    6. How much meat and fresh produce do you consume per day?

27. The patient has a very low platelet count. Which instruction will the nurse give to the UAP about the care of this patient? *(291)*
    1. Always wear a mask to prevent spreading respiratory droplets.
    2. Handle the patient very gently to avoid bruising and injury.
    3. Encourage the patient to take fluids to prevent dehydration.
    4. Assist the patient with hygiene to prevent undue fatigue.

28. An adolescent with hemophilia A wants to participate in a high school sports activity. In consultation with the health care provider, which sport would be the best? *(293)*
    1. Football
    2. Soccer
    3. Wrestling
    4. Golf

29. The nurse reads in the record that the patient has a medical diagnosis of Hodgkin's disease Stage 1. Which sign/symptom would the nurse expect to see? *(299)*
    1. Abnormal single lymph node
    2. Night sweats
    3. Weight loss
    4. Alcohol-induced pain

30. Based on the nurse's knowledge of non-Hodgkin's disease, what does the nurse consider when planning care for the patient who has recently started treatment? (Select all that apply.) *(301)*
    1. Pain is likely to be localized in the spine and increased with movement.
    2. Disease is likely to be widespread and most body systems are affected.
    3. Patient could have side effects from chemotherapy.
    4. Patient and/or family may need support because prognosis is poor.
    5. Total assistance for ADLs is likely to be needed.

CRITICAL THINKING ACTIVITIES

Activity 1

31. A 63-year-old patient is seen with complaints of her "heart racing," nausea, sore tongue, and difficulty swallowing. Upon oral examination, her tongue is smooth and erythematous. *(275, 276)*

    a. What medical diagnosis would a nurse anticipate? _____

    b. What diagnostic tests will support this suspicion? _____

    _____

    c. What treatment options are available for this patient? _____

    _____

    d. After completing 2 months of treatment, the patient states she is feeling well and now plans to discontinue the treatments. How should the nurse respond to the patient?

    _____

    _____

Activity 2

32. A 32-year-old female patient comes for care with complaints of fatigue, dizziness, and pallor. Her history includes childbirth 3 months ago, a subgastrectomy 3 years ago, and hernia repair 18 months ago. Her Hgb level is 10 g/dL. *(279, 280)*

    a. Based on the nurse's knowledge, what is the anticipated medical diagnosis? _____

    _____

    b. What risk factors does this patient have that support development of this disorder? _____

    _____

    _____

c. Identify other signs and symptoms that may accompany this disorder. _____

_____

_____

d. Discuss six considerations for the administration of iron. _____

_____

_____

Activity 3

33. The nurse is caring for an older adult patient who reports bone pain that increases with movement. The medical diagnosis is multiple myeloma.

a. Discuss the benefits of ambulation and fluid for this patient. *(296, 297)*_____

_____

_____

b. What can the nurse do to encourage the patient to walk if he says that moving increases the pain? *(296, 297)*

_____

_____

_____

Activity 4

34. Use the nursing process and indicate general care for patients with disorders of the hematologic and lymphatic systems. *(302, 303)*

Assessment	
Nursing diagnoses	
Planning	
Implementation	
Evaluation	

Care of the Patient with a Cardiovascular or a Peripheral Vascular Disorder

chapter

8

Answer Key: Textbook page references are provided as a guide for answering these questions. A complete Answer Key is provided in your Additional Learning Resources on Evolve.

TRACING A DROP OF BLOOD

1. Directions: Trace a drop of blood around the systemic circulatory system. Start at the superior or inferior vena cava and identify the names of the blood vessels, the chambers of the heart, and the valves of the heart. End with the drop of blood at the aorta. *(312)*

   Superior or inferior vena cava →

   _____ → _____ →

   _____ → _____ →

   _____ → _____ →

   _____ → _____ →

   _____ → _____ →

   _____ → Aorta.

2. Directions: Identify the impulse pattern of the electrical conduction system of the heart. Start at the SA node. *(310)*

   SA node →

   _____ →_____ →

   _____ →_____

FIGURE LABELING

3. Directions: Label each of the coronary vessels that supply blood to the heart. *(310)*

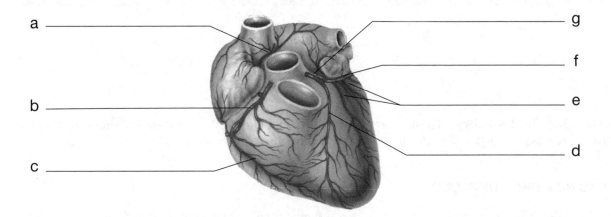

MATCHING

Directions: Match the term on the left with the explanation to the patient on the right. Record the letter of the correct choice in the space provided.

Term	Explanation to the Patient
_____ 4. Aneurysm *(367)*	a. An electric shock to your chest; restores your regular heartbeat
_____ 5. Angina pectoris *(327)*	b. Slow, steady heart rate
_____ 6. Arteriosclerosis *(362)*	c. Part of the blood vessel is blocked
_____ 7. Atherosclerosis *(362)*	d. The arteries are thicker and not as stretchy
_____ 8. Bradycardia *(320)*	e. Chest pain and choking sensations that are relieved by nitroglycerin
_____ 9. Cardioversion *(315)*	f. Bulging of an artery, like a tire with a bulge
_____ 10. Coronary artery disease *(326)*	g. Removing the plaques from the inner part of arteries
	h. You do not have enough oxygen in your blood
_____ 11. Defibrillation *(323)*	i. A blood clot or foreign matter travels in the bloodstream
_____ 12. Dysrhythmia *(320)*	j. An abnormal heartbeat
_____ 13. Embolus *(333)*	k. A condition that causes the blood to stop going to the arteries around the heart
_____ 14. Endarterectomy *(365)*	l. In order to breathe, you may have to sit or stand up
_____ 15. Heart failure *(338)*	m. Shocking the heart to stop ventricular fibrillation, which prevents the heart from pumping blood
_____ 16. Hypoxemia *(315)*	n. Fluid is collecting in the lining around the lungs
_____ 17. Intermittent claudication *(356)*	o. You have too many red blood cells in your blood
	p. Your heart is not pumping effectively, causing fluid to settle in the lungs
_____ 18. Ischemia *(327)*	q. The arteries are filling up with plaque and beginning to close
_____ 19. Myocardial infarction *(333)*	r. The heart cannot pump correctly
_____ 20. Occlusion *(333)*	s. Very fast heart rate that is steady
_____ 21. Orthopnea *(346)*	t. Cramps and weakness in your legs caused by decreased blood flow to your muscles
_____ 22. Peripheral *(355)*	u. A body part or organ is not getting enough blood, thus causin pain
_____ 23. Pleural effusion *(312)*	v. The heart is being damaged by the lack of blood
_____ 24. Polycythemia *(315)*	w. Arms and legs
_____ 25. Pulmonary edema *(344)*	
_____ 26. Tachycardia *(320)*	

FILL-IN-THE-BLANK SENTENCES

Directions: Complete each sentence by filling in the blank with the correct word or phrase.

27. For many years, creatine phosphokinase (CK-MB) was the gold standard for the diagnosis of myocardial infarction, but now _____ are preferred. *(316)*

28. Some researchers believe that elevated levels of homocysteine can be treated by administration of vitamins _____, _____, and _____. *(317)*

29. Older Americans should have their cholesterol tested once every _____ years. *(317)*

30. _____ and _____ have been identified as good forms of exercise to decrease the risk of developing cardiovascular disease. *(319)*

31. _____ is pain (usually in the calves) brought on by exercise and relieved by rest. *(356)*

32. For Buerger's disease, the most important patient behavior is _____. *(369)*

MULTIPLE CHOICE

Directions: Select the best answer(s) for each of the following questions.

33. The nurse is caring for a patient who is on anticoagulant therapy. Which laboratory values are the most important to monitor? *(315)*
    1. Prothrombin time, International Normalized Ratio, and partial thromboplastin time
    2. Blood glucose, potassium, sodium, calcium, and magnesium
    3. Enzyme creatine kinase, creatine phosphokinase, and myoglobin
    4. B-type natriuretic peptide and troponins 1 and 2

34. Laboratory results show a low hemoglobin for a patient diagnosed with myocardial infarction. What is the first therapy that the nurse would ensure to address this laboratory result? *(337)*
    1. Obtain an order for an intramuscular iron supplement.
    2. Help the patient to order an iron-rich meal tray.
    3. Obtain an order for type and cross for blood transfusion.
    4. Check to see that oxygen is delivered as ordered.

35. The nurse is planning care for several patients who are scheduled to have diagnostic testing for cardiac disorders. Which patient will require postprocedural checks for peripheral pulses, color, and sensation of the extremity every 15 minutes for 1 hour? *(312)*
    1. Needs cardiac catheterization to diagnose extent of atherosclerotic heart disease
    2. Is scheduled for electrocardiogram to identify specific cardiac dysrhythmias
    3. Requires chemically induced stress electrocardiogram for poor exercise tolerance
    4. Must have positron emission tomography because of coronary artery disease

36. The nurse is discussing modifiable risk factors for cardiovascular disease with a 23-year-old patient who is currently asymptomatic. What does the nurse recommend? *(318)*
    1. Find out if any first-degree relatives had cardiovascular problems before 50 years of age.
    2. Stop smoking or consider greatly reducing the number of cigarettes smoked per day.
    3. Ask your health care provider for a cholesterol-lowering drug, such as simvastatin (Zocor).
    4. Monitor weight and calorie intake to maintain a body mass index of 30.

37. During a discharge teaching session, the patient voices concern about why her risk of heart disease is elevated simply because she has a history of diabetes mellitus. What is the best explanation to give to the patient? *(319)*
    1. Fluctuating insulin levels cause vasoconstriction.
    2. Elevated blood glucose levels contribute to arterial damage.
    3. Diabetics are obese and thus at higher risk.
    4. Risk for heart disease is not higher for people with diabetes.

38. Which psychosocial behaviors are more likely to be associated with increased cardiovascular symptoms? *(320)*
    1. Frequently in a hurry and easily irritated
    2. Easygoing and usually enjoys life
    3. Neat, organized, and pays attention to detail
    4. Pessimistic and generally expresses negativity

39. The patient's cardiac monitor shows a regular rhythm with a rate of 65 beats/min, P waves precede each QRS complex, QRS complexes are symmetrical and regularly spaced, and a normal T wave shows repolarization. What is the nurse's interpretation of monitor display? *(320)*
    1. Vital signs should be immediately assessed.
    2. The monitor indicates a normal sinus rhythm.
    3. The monitor is showing a benign dysrhythmia.
    4. The patient should be assessed for chest pain.

40. The patient experiences dizziness and lightheadedness while trying to pass a bowel movement. An immediate pulse check shows 45 beats/min that rapidly recovers to a regular rate of 70. What is the most probable cause of this episode of sinus bradycardia? *(320)*
    1. Digitalis toxicity
    2. Endocrine disturbance
    3. Intracranial tumor
    4. Vagal stimulation

41. For which dysrhythmia would a pacemaker mostly likely be necessary? *(326)*
    1. Sinus tachycardia
    2. Premature ventricular contractions
    3. Third-degree heart block
    4. Atrial fibrillation

42. The patient who had a myocardial infarction 2 weeks ago is now having frequent episodes of ventricular tachycardia. For this patient, what is the clinical significance of this dysrhythmia? *(322)*
    1. Warning sign for ventricular fibrillation
    2. Expected finding at this stage
    3. Reaction to a beta-adrenergic blocker
    4. Treatment is given only for symptoms

43. The patient is on the cardiac monitor undergoing a diagnostic procedure. Suddenly, the health care provider says, "The patient is having ventricular fibrillation." Which piece of equipment is the most vital? *(323)*
    1. Temporary pacemaker
    2. Defibrillator
    3. Bag-valve-mask
    4. Crash cart

44. A patient is being discharged after receiving a permanent pacemaker. What is the best rationale to give to the patient about refraining from sports such as tennis, swimming, golf, and weight-lifting for the first 6-8 weeks? *(326)*
    1. "First, you have to be able to climb at least two flights of stairs."
    2. "Active sports will interfere with the pacemaker's fixed mode."
    3. "These sports are too strenuous and rapidly increase the heart rate."
    4. "The arm on the pacemaker side should not be lifted over the head."

45. The patient had a percutaneous transluminal coronary angioplasty with stent placement. What type of medication is the patient most likely to be prescribed for at least 3 months? *(330)*
    1. Digitalis preparation
    2. Diuretic
    3. Opioid pain medication
    4. Anticoagulant

46. Which instruction would the nurse give to the patient for self-administration of nitrate medications? *(332)*
    1. Refrigerate the oral tablets and nitroglycerin patches until use.
    2. Apply patches in the morning and remove them at bedtime.
    3. A burning sensation on the tongue indicates an allergic reaction.
    4. Pain relief should occur after a minimum of two doses.

47. For a patient with myocardial infarction, what symptom is the most important? *(333)*
    1. Diaphoresis
    2. Palpitations
    3. Pain
    4. Shortness of breath

48. A 63-year-old patient presents with fever, increased pulse, epistaxis, and joint involvement. Heart murmurs are auscultated. The patient has a history of inadequately treated childhood group A β-hemolytic streptococci pharyngitis. These findings and history are consistent with which medical diagnosis? *(349)*
    1. Cardiomyopathy
    2. Angina
    3. Left-sided heart block
    4. Rheumatic heart disease

49. A neighbor tells the nurse that he has indigestion that has lasted 60 minutes. He tried "taking nitroglycerin, but that didn't help." What should the nurse do first? *(329)*
    1. Tell the neighbor to take an aspirin and then drive to the emergency department.
    2. Stay with the neighbor, assist him to remain calm, and call 911.
    3. Assess the neighbor's use of nitroglycerin and assess for other symptoms.
    4. Phone the neighbor's health care provider and ask for recommendations.

50. The health care provider is considering tissue plasminogen activator (TPA) for a patient who is having an acute myocardial infarction. The wife suddenly rushes to the nurse and says, "We forgot to tell you something." Which disclosure is a contraindication for TPA? *(336)*
    1. "My husband is a Jehovah's Witness."
    2. "My husband recently had a head injury."
    3. "He forgot to take his insulin this morning."
    4. "He had a small heart attack last year."

51. The nurse is caring for a patient who is 40 hours post–myocardial infarction. Which instruction should be given to the UAP? *(337)*
    1. Assist the patient to ambulate in the hall three times.
    2. Check to see if the patient is too tired to get up.
    3. Encourage the patient to independently get out of bed.
    4. Help the patient get to the commode chair.

52. What is the best method to help a patient comply with dietary restrictions associated with atherosclerotic heart disease? *(339)*
    1. Tell him to avoid all foods that are high in fats.
    2. Remind him that total fat intake is 35-40% of total caloric intake.
    3. Tell him to eat 10-15 grams of soluble fiber every day.
    4. Teach him how to read the nutritional labels on food products.

53. The nurse is caring for a patient who has right ventricular heart failure. After therapy, the nurse sees that the patient has lost 5 pounds of weight. Assuming that all the weight represents fluid loss, how much fluid has the patient lost? _____ L *(339)*

54. The patient with a history of heart failure tells the home health nurse, "Every night I sleep in this recliner chair. I feel better if I sleep with my head up." What will the nurse assess first? *(340)*
    1. Check for dependent edema in the lower extremities.
    2. Look at accessibility to the bedroom and bathroom.
    3. Assess ability to independently move and ambulate.
    4. Ask about compliance with low-sodium, low-fat diet.

55. The nurse is supervising a nursing student who must administer digoxin to a patient. The nurse would intervene if the student performs which action? *(344)*
    1. Stops to check the potassium level before administering the drug
    2. Asks the patient if he has any questions or concerns about the drug
    3. Tells the patient that his pulse is 55 beats/min and prepares to administer the drug
    4. Checks to see if the drug causes any interactions with other prescribed drugs

56. The patient arrives in the emergency department with severe dyspnea, agitation, cyanosis, audible wheezes, and a cough with blood-tinged sputum. What is the priority nursing action? *(346, 347)*
    1. Obtain a blood sample for arterial blood gases
    2. Administer oxygen
    3. Auscultate lung sounds
    4. Establish a peripheral IV

57. The nurse is caring for a patient with valvular heart disease. Which task could be assigned to the UAP? *(348)*
    1. Identifying ADLs that cause fatigue
    2. Check meal trays for high-sodium foods
    3. Weigh the patient at the same time every day
    4. Explain the plan for rest periods

58. Which disorder of the cardiovascular system places the patient at highest risk for the potentially life-threatening condition of cardiac tamponade? *(350)*
    1. Pericarditis
    2. Valvular heart disease
    3. Buerger's disease
    4. Endocarditis

59. Which sign/symptom indicates to the nurse that a patient with endocarditis is experiencing a serious and common complication of the disease? *(352)*
    1. Fever and chills
    2. Joint pains and aches
    3. Sudden shortness of breath
    4. Petechiae on neck and chest

60. The nurse sees an elderly woman sitting in the waiting room and she is crying, "My granddaughter was just diagnosed with infective endocarditis. Those patients always die within a year." What should the nurse say first to comfort the grandmother? *(353)*
    1. "Surgical procedures can repair the diseased valves."
    2. "These days, intensive antibiotic therapy cures 90% of patients."
    3. "If she is able to rest her heart, she will probably be okay."
    4. "We will do everything we can to take care of her."

61. Which patient should be counseled about the risk of cardiomyopathy related to lifestyle choices? *(353)*
    1. High-risk sexual behavior
    2. Poor intake of dietary fiber
    3. Use of "crack" cocaine
    4. Social consumption of alcohol

62. The patient had a recent cardiac transplant. Which intervention is required for posttransplant care? *(354)*
    1. Immunosuppressive therapy
    2. Pericardiocentesis
    3. Percutaneous transluminal angioplasty
    4. Contact isolation

63. What treatments and/or advice are given to patients who are prehypertensive? *(359)*
    1. Diuretics and low-sodium diet
    2. Beta-adrenergic blockers and weight loss
    3. Angiotensin II receptor blockers and low-fat diet
    4. Lifestyle change and routine health appointments

64. The nurse is caring for a patient who has peripheral arterial disease with burning pain that occurs at rest in the right leg. For the nursing diagnosis of Ineffective Tissue Perfusion related to decreased arterial blood flow, which intervention will the nurse use? *(364)*
    1. Elevate the leg on a pillow
    2. Use a covered ice compress
    3. Place the leg in a dependent position
    4. Encourage aerobic exercise for circulation

65. A patient receives a prescription for anticoagulant medication for treatment of arterial emboli. What dietary information should the nurse give? *(366)*
    1. Do not increase intake of dark-green vegetables because of vitamin K.
    2. Take extra dairy products to ensure calcium intake and vitamin D.
    3. Eat fruits such as citrus and bananas that provide potassium.
    4. Avoid eating saturated fats by limiting use of butter, oils, and red meats.

66. The nurse is monitoring a patient who is waiting for diagnostic testing to determine if he has an aortic aneurysm. The patient suddenly reports severe chest pain. He becomes pale, weak, and confused. His pulse is 130 beats/min and blood pressure is 85/50 mm Hg. What should the nurse do first? *(368)*
    1. Call the health care provider
    2. Put the patient in a supine position
    3. Assess pain and give opioid medication
    4. Establish a patent peripheral IV

67. The nurse is caring for a postsurgical patient. Which intervention is the most important in preventing deep vein thrombosis in the legs? *(374)*
    1. Applying elastic compression stockings
    2. Elevating the lower extremities
    3. Ensuring early ambulation and mobility
    4. Measuring the calf circumference daily

CRITICAL THINKING ACTIVITIES

Activity 1

68. A 56-year-old man arrives in the emergency department seeking care. He is complaining of crushing chest pain. The pain is radiating down his left shoulder and arm. The patient, who has a history of angina, reports the pain is more severe and has lasted longer than a typical angina episode. *(333-337)*

    a. What does the nurse anticipate this patient's medical diagnosis will be? _____

       _____

    b. Discuss the pathology of this type of occurrence. _____

       _____

    c. During the medical diagnostic workup of this patient, what tests are likely to be ordered?

       _____

       _____

    d. What are the goals of the medical management of this patient? _____

       _____

       _____

    e. Identify four nursing interventions for this patient's care. _____

       _____

       _____

Activity 2

69. A 43-year-old Native American woman presents with complaints of "heaviness in her chest." She reports that it radiates down her left inner arm. Her medical history includes childbirth, pancreatitis, and hypertension. The medical diagnosis of angina is made. *(327-329)*

    a. What risk factors for heart disease does the patient have? _____

       _____

       _____

    b. What medications are used to treat angina? _____

       _____

    c. The patient asks the nurse, "What has caused this to happen?" How will the nurse respond to her inquiry?

       _____

Activity 3

70. A home health nurse is caring for a 73-year-old man who has heart failure. He has been hospitalized twice for exacerbations, but is currently stable and able to live independently in his own home.

   a. What changes related to aging would the nurse expect to find for this patient's cardiac system? *(317, 355)*

   _____

   _____

   b. What are common signs and symptoms of heart failure? *(338, 339)* _____

   _____

   _____

   c. Identify medication classes that are used in the medical management of heart failure. *(341-343)*

   _____

   _____

   d. Discuss patient teaching points for heart failure. *(344)* _____

   _____

   _____

Activity 4

71. The nurse is working in an ambulatory walk-in clinic in an urban area. Many of the patients are homeless and the clinic staff sees many patients who have venous stasis ulcers.

   a. What is the pathophysiology of stasis ulcers and why are the homeless at particular risk for this disorder? *(374)*

   _____

   b. Describe how the nurse would use PATCHES to assess venous disorders. *(356)* _____

   _____

   _____

   _____

   c. Identify the signs and symptoms of venous stasis ulcers. *(374)* _____

   _____

   _____

   d. Review the treatment options available for venous stasis ulcers and suggest how the nurse can assist homeless patients with these options. *(375, 376)*

   _____

   _____

Activity 5

72. Check the cupboards of an elderly relative or patient (or your own cupboards) and read nutritional labels on packages. Determine if a typical day's use of the products on the shelf would meet the nutritional restrictions for someone on a cardioprotective diet. (Don't forget to check condiments, if they are likely to be included in daily use.) Record your findings and the recommendations that you would make about the choice of food products. *(339)*

_____

_____

_____

_____

_____

_____

_____

_____

Care of the Patient with a Respiratory Disorder

chapter

9

Answer Key: Textbook page references are provided as a guide for answering these questions. A complete Answer Key is provided in your Additional Learning Resources on Evolve.

MATCHING

Medication Used for Respiratory Disorders

Directions: Match the medication used for a respiratory disorder on the left to the associated characteristic (action, side effect, or nursing implication) on the right. Indicate your answers in the spaces provided. (411, 412)

Medication	Actions, Side Effects, or Nursing Implications
_____ 1. Acetylcysteine (Mucomyst)	a. Vasoconstrictor, used for nasal congestion
_____ 2. Salmeterol (Serevent)	b. Beta$_1$- and beta$_2$-receptor agonist; could cause tachycardia, palpitations, angina, chest pain, myocardial infarction (MI), dysrhythmias, hypertension, restlessness, agitation, anxiety
_____ 3. Prednisone (Deltasone)	c. Bronchodilator; can cause anxiety, restlessness, insomnia, headache, seizures, tachycardia, dysrhythmias
_____ 4. Epinephrine (Adrenalin)	d. Mucolytic agent; also used as antidote in acetaminophen overdose
_____ 5. Ethambutol (Myambutol)	e. Used in prevention of exercise-induced asthma
_____ 6. Isoniazid (INH) (Nydrazid)	f. Antiinflammatory agent ; do not discontinue medication abruptly; dosage must be tapered slowly
_____ 7. Oxymetazoline (Afrin)	g. Antitubercular agent; requires baseline visual examination at start of therapy
_____ 8. Theophylline (Theo-Dur)	h. Antitubercular agent; monitor liver function tests
_____ 9. Potassium iodide	i. For long-term treatment of asthma
_____ 10. Zafirlukast (Accolate)	j. Expectorant, mucokinetic agent; could cause hyperkalemia

FILL-IN-THE-BLANK SENTENCES

Directions: Complete each sentence by filling in the blank with the correct word or phrase.

11. Carbon dioxide and oxygen diffuse between blood and lung _____ and alveolar air. *(386)*

12. At rest, the normal inspiration lasts about _____ seconds and expiration about _____ seconds. *(386)*

13. When stimulated by increasing levels of blood _____, decreasing levels of blood _____, or increasing blood acidity, the chemoreceptors send nerve impulses to the respiratory centers, which in turn modify respiratory rates. *(386)*

14. The pco_2 level is _____ in primary respiratory acidosis and _____ in primary respiratory alkalosis. *(391)*

15. _____ are tissue growths on the nasal tissues that are frequently caused by prolonged sinus inflammation. *(394)*

TRUE OR FALSE

Directions: Write T for true or F for false in the blanks provided.

_____   16.   Aspirated foreign bodies are more likely to lodge in the left main stem bronchus. *(384)*

_____   17.   Lung cancer is now the leading cause of death from cancer for men only. *(424)*

_____   18.   Cigarette smoking is by far the most common cause of emphysema and chronic bronchitis. *(433)*

_____   19.   In general, infants and young children with pulmonary tuberculosis (TB) do not require isolation precautions because they rarely cough and their bronchial secretions contain few acid-fast bacilli (AFB) compared with adults with pulmonary TB. *(411)*

TABLE ACTIVITY

20. Directions: Complete the table by filling in the normal values for an arterial blood gas. *(391)*

pH:	
$Paco_2$:	
Pao_2:	
HCO_3^-:	
Sao_2:	

MULTIPLE CHOICE

Directions: Select the best answer(s) for each of the following questions.

21. The patient had a permanent tracheostomy placed several months ago. The nurse will design interventions for the patient's inability to: *(399)*
    1. breathe independently and safely.
    2. secrete adequate amounts of mucus.
    3. physiologically produce normal speech.
    4. swallow without choking or gagging.

22. A patient with a chronic lung disorder comes to the clinic and tells the nurse, "I feel like I am getting sick again." What questions would the nurse ask? (Select all that apply.) *(386, 387)*
    1. "How's your breathing? Can you describe it?"
    2. "Are you coughing? Can you describe the cough?"
    3. "When did you first notice the worsening of symptoms?"
    4. "What were your last arterial blood gas results?"
    5. "Do you use oxygen at home? If so, does it help?"
    6. "Have you noticed a change in your ability to do routine activities?"

23. The patient arrives at the emergency department and displays significant respiratory distress. Which objective finding is generally regarded as a late sign of respiratory distress? *(387)*
    1. Shows increased respiratory rate
    2. Has adventitious breath sounds
    3. Assumes orthopneic position
    4. Demonstrates flaring of nostrils

24. A patient was brought to the emergency department because he was involved in a motor vehicle accident. The patient shows mild respiratory distress and expansion of the right side of the chest is decreased compared to the left. The history and data are indicative of which disorder? *(423)*
    1. Pleural effusion
    2. Pneumothorax
    3. Empyema
    4. Pulmonary edema

25. Which patient has the greatest need for a helical computed tomography scan, which is considered a new and improved technology? *(429)*
    1. A disoriented elderly man who may have a pulmonary embolus
    2. A toddler who might have swallowed a metallic foreign body
    3. A patient who requires a sample of lymph node tissue for biopsy
    4. A patient who was exposed to tuberculosis several decades ago

26. The nurse is caring for a patient who had a bronchoscopy. Which task can be delegated to the UAP? *(389)*
    1. Give clear fluids after checking for the gag reflex.
    2. Assist the patient to a semi-Fowler's position.
    3. Report signs of laryngeal edema, such as stridor.
    4. Check sputum for signs of hemorrhage.

27. The patient needs a thoracentesis for therapeutic reasons. Which position should the nurse help the patient to assume for the procedure? *(390)*
    1. Seated on the bed; head and arms resting on a pillow placed on an overbed table
    2. Placed in a supine position with the anterior-lateral chest draped for ready access
    3. Positioned in a recumbent prone position with head resting on forearms and hands
    4. Situated in a side-lying position on affected side and uncovered to the waist

28. The nurse hears in change of shift report that 1500 mL of fluid was removed during the therapeutic thoracentesis procedure. What is the most important intervention that the nurse will plan to do? *(390)*
    1. Perform routine postprocedure assessments.
    2. Increase the fluid intake to compensate for the loss.
    3. Watch for signs and symptoms of pulmonary edema.
    4. Follow up to get the results of the fluid specimen.

29. What special consideration is needed for an arterial blood gas for a patient who is taking warfarin (Coumadin)? *(429)*
    1. The dietary therapy associated with the drug is likely to alter the results.
    2. The drug increases fragility of the vessels, so the specimen is hard to obtain.
    3. The drug alters the amount of oxygen that hemoglobin can carry.
    4. The clotting times are longer than normal, so pressure is held for 20 minutes on the puncture site.

30. The nursing student uses an automatic blood pressure cuff to take vital signs. To be efficient, the student simultaneously attaches the pulse oximeter to the patient's same hand. The pulse oximeter reading is below 90%. What should the student do first? *(392)*
    1. Report the findings to the nurse or instructor.
    2. Redo the pulse oximeter reading on the other hand.
    3. Assess the patient for shortness of breath.
    4. Document the finding in the patient's record.

31. A patient was treated for epistaxis with nasal packing saturated with 1:1000 epinephrine. During the postprocedure assessment, the nurse notices that the patient swallows frequently. Which question should the nurse ask? *(393)*
    1. Does your throat feel swollen or painful?
    2. Would you like some cool fluids to drink?
    3. Is blood running down the back of your throat?
    4. Do you taste the epinephrine in the back of the throat?

32. What is likely to be included in the discharge instructions for a patient who was treated for epistaxis? (Select all that apply.) *(394)*
    1. Use a vaporizer.
    2. Use saline nose drops.
    3. Apply nasal lubricants.
    4. Take aspirin for pain as needed.
    5. Vigorously blow to remove clots.
    6. Avoid inserting foreign objects into nose.

33. What is the nurse's role in allergy testing? *(395)*
    1. Uses a lancet to prick the skin with different allergens
    2. Evaluates the response to different allergens
    3. Advises the patient about allergens to avoid
    4. Determines schedule for retesting questionable allergens

34. The nurse is eating in a restaurant. At a nearby table, several men are talking, laughing, drinking alcohol, and eating steak. Suddenly, the nurse hears, "Heh! Are you all right?" Which behavior signals a need to intervene for choking? *(397)*
    1. Vigorous coughing
    2. Running from the room
    3. Hand over throat
    4. Waving hands frantically

35. A patient is diagnosed with viral laryngitis. Which discharge instruction is the most important to relieve the inflammation and edema of the vocal cords? *(403)*
    1. Use a mild analgesic, such as acetaminophen for pain.
    2. Complete the full course of antibiotics.
    3. Rest the voice; communicate with gestures or by writing.
    4. Suck on throat lozenges to promote comfort.

36. The nurse is performing a rapid strep screen. What is the rationale for obtaining two throat swabs? *(403)*
    1. The first swab is likely to be contaminated, so a backup swab is needed.
    2. If the rapid strep test is negative, the second swab is sent for culture.
    3. The second swab is given to the patient, in case the rapid strep is positive.
    4. The first and second swabs are grown in different types of culture media.

37. A patient comes to the clinic and reports decreased appetite, generalized malaise, and a decreased sense of smell. Gentle palpation over the sinus area elicits pain. Which piece of equipment should the nurse prepare so the health care provider can do some diagnostic testing during the physical examination? *(404)*
    1. Tongue blade
    2. Percussion hammer
    3. Penlight
    4. Cotton-tipped applicator

38. A patient is diagnosed with acute bronchitis. Although the patient is instructed to increase fluids to 3000-4000 mL per day, which fluid is specifically not recommended because of the respiratory condition? *(406)*
    1. Coffee
    2. Soda
    3. Orange juice
    4. Milk

39. What is the primary problem for the health care team in identifying respiratory disorders such as Legionnaires' disease, severe acute respiratory syndrome, and anthrax? *(406-408)*
    1. They are agents used in global germ warfare.
    2. The percentage of morbidity and mortality is high.
    3. They require isolation because transmission is airborne.
    4. At first, symptoms are similar to other respiratory disorders.

40. What is the biggest problem for patients who are being treated for tuberculosis? *(414)*
    1. All the patient's contacts have to be identified and treated.
    2. Infection control measures are complex and expensive.
    3. Many have rapid disease progression with mortality rates up to 89%.
    4. Drug therapy lasts 6 to 9 months and about 50% are noncompliant.

41. A patient recently diagnosed with peripherally located lung cancer reports he is experiencing severe chest pain. Based on the nurse's knowledge of the pathophysiology of this pain, which therapy does the nurse anticipate? *(419, 425)*
    1. Bronchodilators
    2. Thoracentesis
    3. Mechanical ventilation
    4. Corticosteroids

42. The patient is diagnosed with pleurisy. During auscultation of the lungs, what is the nurse most likely to hear? *(387)*
    1. Interrupted crackling or bubbling sounds more common on inspiration
    2. Deep, loud, low, coarse sound (like a snore) during inspiration or expiration
    3. Dry, creaking, grating, with a machinelike quality loudest over anterior chest
    4. High-pitched, musical, whistlelike sound during inspiration or expiration

43. A patient being treated for atelectasis has been prescribed acetylcysteine (Mucomyst). What is the purpose of this medication? *(422)*
    1. Reduce the risk of infection
    2. Dilate the bronchioles
    3. Enhance the cough reflex
    4. Reduce viscosity of secretions

44. For a patient with a chest tube, which task could be delegated to the UAP? *(420)*
    1. Assist to ambulate with water-seal below the level of the chest.
    2. Check to make sure that all connections are secure and intact.
    3. Observe for and report hypoventilation or increased dyspnea.
    4. Assess quantity and quality of drainage in the collection chamber.

45. The nurse is reviewing the admission orders for a patient who was stabilized in the emergency department and then admitted for a diagnosis of pulmonary edema. Which order is the nurse most likely to question? *(427)*
    1. Oxygen 2 liters per nasal cannula
    2. Notify provider with all blood gas results
    3. IV normal saline at 250 mL per hour
    4. Place on telemetry monitor

46. A patient is admitted for a deep vein thrombosis in the left leg. He is in good spirits during the AM assessment, but later in day he reports feeling mildly short of breath with a sense of impending doom. What should the nurse do first? *(429)*
    1. Obtain an order for an arterial blood gas.
    2. Check the vital signs and pulse oximeter reading.
    3. Assess the left leg for warmth, redness, or swelling.
    4. Alert the RN about possible pulmonary embolus.

47. Which patient is most likely to develop acute respiratory distress syndrome (ARDS)? *(431, 432)*
    1. Was diagnosed and treated for sepsis 5 days ago
    2. Had direct trauma to chest during a fight 10 days ago
    3. Has a history of chronic obstructive pulmonary disease
    4. Has been treated for asthma since early childhood

48. Which instruction would the nurse give to the UAP related to assisting the patient who has emphysema with ADLs? *(434)*
    1. Divide hygienic care into short sessions with 90 minutes of rest between.
    2. Defer the hygienic care until the patient has better activity tolerance.
    3. Assess the patient's response to ambulating and shorten walks accordingly.
    4. Perform range-of-motion exercises, unless the patient declines them.

49. For a patient with chronic bronchitis, what is the physiologic cause of polycythemia? *(434)*
    1. Medication side effect
    2. Dehydration and fluid shifting
    3. Nutritional deficiency
    4. Compensation for chronic hypoxemia

50. For a patient with newly diagnosed asthma, what is the rationale for conducting an assessment of the home environment? *(440)*
    1. Determine if the patient will have activity intolerance related to design of house
    2. Assess the safety of the environment related to the use of home oxygen
    3. Identify stimulants or allergens that are triggering the asthma attacks
    4. Evaluate the need for home health care to accomplish activities of daily living

CRITICAL THINKING ACTIVITIES

Activity 1

51. A 34-year-old man comes to the health care provider's office seeking care. He is complaining of fatigue and headaches in the morning. The nurse's assessment reveals he is 5'9" and weighs 293 pounds. His blood pressure is 155/92 mm Hg. His health history reveals elevated blood pressure, hernia repair, appendectomy, and recent injuries suffered from a motor vehicle accident after falling asleep while driving. During the interview, his wife states he should never be tired because he snores so loudly at night that she is the one who is kept awake. *(396, 397)*

    a. Based on the nurse's knowledge, what medical diagnosis is anticipated?_____

    _____

    b. What risk factors and elements of the patient's personal history support this diagnosis? _____

    _____

    _____

    _____

    c. Discuss the medical management of this condition. _____

    _____

    _____

    _____

    _____

Activity 2

52. A 72-year-old man is transferred from the nursing home to the hospital with a diagnosis of viral pneumonia. *(414-418)*

    a.   What signs and symptoms are associated with this type of pneumonia? _____

    _____

    _____

    b.   What diagnostic tests can the nurse expect to be completed for this patient? _____

    _____

    _____

    c.   What types of medications may be prescribed for this patient?_____

    _____

    _____

    d.   Identify nursing assessments that should be performed for this patient._____

    _____

    _____

Activity 3

53. Discuss factors that may influence medication compliance for tuberculosis patients and suggest interventions to increase compliance. *(411-414)*

    _____

    _____

    _____

    _____

    _____

    _____

    _____

    _____

    _____

    _____

    _____

    _____

Activity 4

54. The nurse has arrived on the nursing unit and found that the patient has a closed chest drainage system. *(421)*

   a.   What nursing assessments should be performed for this patient? _____

   _____

   _____

   b.   How should the tubing and the chest drainage system be positioned? _____

   _____

   _____

   c.   What is indicated if there is no tidaling (air bubbling) noted in the water seal chamber?_____

   _____

   _____

   d.   What does constant bubbling in the water seal chamber indicate? _____

   _____

   _____

Care of the Patient with a Urinary Disorder

chapter
10

Answer Key: Textbook page references are provided as a guide for answering these questions. A complete Answer Key is provided in your Additional Learning Resources on Evolve.

WORD SCRAMBLE

Directions: Unscramble the words that are related to pathology of the urinary system and then match the term to the correct definition or characteristic listed below.

Scrambled Term	Unscrambled Term	Definition or Characteristic
1. riaanu *(455)*		
2. aimetoza *(468)*		
3. terbaciuria *(464)*		
4. sislydiahemo *(489)*		
5. suriady *(453)*		
6. airutameh *(464)*		
7. urianoct *(464)*		
8. guriailo *(476)*		
9. dyniaprostato *(467)*		
10. thiasisuro *(471)*		

Definition or characteristic of terms related to pathology of the urinary system
a. Retention of excessive amounts of nitrogenous compounds in the blood
b. Blood in the urine
c. Excessive urination at night
d. Urinary output of less than 100 mL/day
e. Painful or difficult urination
f. Requires access to the circulatory system to route blood through the artificial kidney
g. Formation of urinary calculi
h. Decreased urinary output, less than 500 mL in 24 hours
i. Bacteria in urine
j. Pain in the prostate gland

SHORT ANSWERS

Directions: Using your own words, answer each question in the space provided.

11. What are the three major functions of the nephron? *(447)*

    a. _____

    b. _____

    c. _____

12. Summarize the three phases of urine formation. *(448)*

    a. _____

    b. _____

    c. _____

13. Identify three life span considerations for older adults related to the urinary system. *(450)*

    a. _____

    b. _____

    c. _____

TABLE ACTIVITY

Directions: Complete the table below by supplying the normal range for urinalysis results and identify at least one factor that could influence the results. The first constituent is completed for you. (451)

14. Urinalysis

Constituent	Normal Range	Influencing Factors
Color	Pale yellow to amber	Diabetes insipidus, biliary obstruction, medications, diet
Turbidity		
Odor		
pH		
Specific gravity		
Glucose		
Protein		
Bilirubin		
Hemoglobin		
Ketones		
Red blood cells		
White blood cells		
Casts		
Bacteria		

FIGURE LABELING

15. Directions: Identify the ileal conduit, stoma, and anastomosis on the figure below. *(494)*

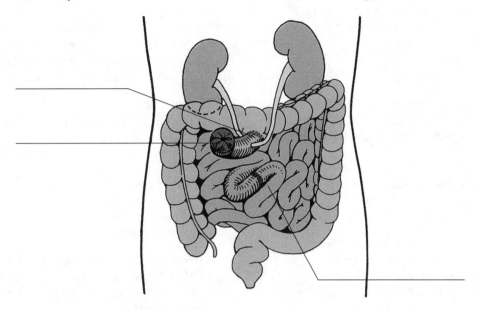

MULTIPLE CHOICE

Directions: Select the best answer(s) for each of the following questions.

16. A patient diagnosed with a urinary tract infection was directed to take sulfamethoxazole-trimethoprim (Bactrim) for 3 days and phenazopyridine (Pyridium) for 2 days. What abnormal finding would be expected to occur in the urine during treatment? *(465)*
    1. An increase in pH
    2. Bright orange color
    3. Increase in leukocytes
    4. Presence of ketones

17. For patients with diabetes mellitus or starvation states, urinalysis will show the abnormal presences of ketones. What is the underlying physiology for this abnormality? *(449)*
    1. Fatty acids are rapidly catabolized.
    2. Glucose is converted to ketones.
    3. Insulin levels are excessive.
    4. Glucose is transformed into fat.

18. Which patient condition is most likely to result in casts in the urine specimen? *(451)*
    1. Type 1 diabetes mellitus
    2. Corticosteroid use
    3. Renal disease
    4. Urinary structure trauma

19. The nurse sees that the urine specific gravity results are 1.00o g/mL. Which patient condition is most likely to result in this abnormal finding? *(452)*
    1. Diabetic ketoacidosis
    2. Hyperemesis gravidarum
    3. Water intoxication
    4. Febrile with poor skin turgor

20. Identify the renal disorders associated with an abnormal elevation in serum creatinine. (Select all that apply.) *(452)*
    1. Prostatitis
    2. Glomerulonephritis
    3. Pyelonephritis
    4. Acute tubular necrosis
    5. Acute renal failure

21. A 49-year-old man's prostate-specific antigen (PSA) result is 9.5 ng/mL. Which condition(s) could be associated with this result? (Select all that apply.) *(452)*
    1. Had a recent prostate biopsy
    2. Could be related to prostate cancer
    3. Suggests urinary tract infection
    4. Indicative of prostatitis
    5. Within normal limits

22. The nurse is planning care for several patients who will have diagnostic testing for urinary disorders. Which procedure is going to require the most time for postprocedural care? *(453)*
    1. Kidney-ureter-bladder radiography
    2. Intravenous pyelogram
    3. Renal angiography
    4. Renal ultrasonography

23. During a urodynamic study, a patient is given bethanechol (Urecholine), a cholinergic drug. What is the expected effect of the medication? *(454)*
    1. Relaxes the patient
    2. Reduces urine production
    3. Stimulates the atonic bladder
    4. Increases the uptake of dye

24. What instructions would the nurse give to the UAP for assisting a patient for the first 24 hours after a renal biopsy? *(454)*
    1. Assist the patient to ambulate to the bathroom.
    2. Ask the patient about dizziness before ambulating.
    3. Withhold all foods and fluids for 24 hours.
    4. Remind the patient about bedrest for 24 hours.

25. The nurse is reviewing medication orders for a patient with advanced end-stage renal disease. The nurse would question the use of which type of medication? *(456)*
    1. Antiemetic
    2. Antipruritic
    3. Vitamin supplement
    4. Osmotic diuretic

26. The nurse is caring for several elderly men who have problems with urinary disorders. Which patient is the best candidate for an external condom? *(458)*
    1. Has Alzheimer's disease and recently pulled out an indwelling catheter
    2. Has urge incontinence and functional incontinence related to a hip fracture
    3. Has a urinary tract infection and is currently taking antibiotics
    4. Has an enlarged prostate and occasionally has trouble starting the stream

27. The UAP tells the nurse that the patient with a urinary catheter has urine output of less than 50 mL/hour. What should the nurse do first? *(477)*
    1. Notify the RN and health care provider.
    2. Ask the UAP to recheck the amount.
    3. Assess the patient for renal failure.
    4. Check the function of the drainage system.

28. The nurse sees that the patient who is being discharged is prescribed spironolactone (Aldactone). Which laboratory result will the nurse verify before the patient goes home? *(456)*
    1. Urinalysis
    2. Potassium level
    3. White cell count
    4. Blood urea nitrogen

29. A patient with benign prostatic hyperplasia (BPH) tells the nurse that he uses over-the-counter medications. Which medication is likely to create additional problems related to the BPH? *(460)*
    1. Acetaminophen (Ibuprofen)
    2. Diphenhydramine (Benadryl)
    3. Vitamin K supplement
    4. Iron supplement

30. Which patient is most likely to benefit from learning about Kegel exercises? *(460)*
    1. Experiences loss of urine during sneezing and lifting
    2. Has urinary retention secondary to chronic infection
    3. Has urge incontinence due to advanced Parkinson's disease
    4. Has a spastic bladder due to upper motor neuron lesion

31. The nurse and UAP are aware that no tension should be placed on urinary catheters; however the nurse should reinforce this principle for which patient? *(481)*
    1. Has a suprapubic catheter for long-term management
    2. Has a three-way catheter for continuous bladder irrigation
    3. Has a Foley catheter after reconstruction of urethra
    4. Has a catheter and urometer for hourly measurements

32. For patients with nephrotic syndrome, which signs/symptoms is the nurse most likely to observe? *(482)*
    1. Periorbital edema, pitting edema in legs, and crackles in lungs
    2. Sore throat or skin infection with fever and malaise
    3. Burning with urination, low back pain, hematuria, and fatigue
    4. Dysuria, weak stream, and increasing pain with bladder distention

33. The patient with acute glomerulonephritis is placed on bedrest. Which vital sign is of primary interest as an indicator of the success of the therapy? *(483)*
    1. Temperature
    2. Pulse rate
    3. Respiratory rate
    4. Blood pressure

34. What is an early indicator of kidney failure that should be routinely checked for patients who are at high risk? *(484)*
    1. Residual urine
    2. Albumin in the urine
    3. Ketones in the urine
    4. Prostate-specific antigen

35. What does the nurse do to assess the function of an arteriovenous fistula after a dialysis treatment? *(489)*
    1. Flush with saline using strict aseptic technique.
    2. Palpate a thrill and auscultate for a bruit.
    3. Assess the distal pulses and check for sensation.
    4. Ask the patient about pain or discomfort at the site.

CRITICAL THINKING ACTIVITIES

Activity 1

36. A 42-year-old patient is admitted to the unit with a diagnosis of pyelonephritis. As the nurse collects data, she reveals a history of diabetes mellitus, and frequent urinary tract infections. *(468, 469)*

    a. What signs and symptoms would the nurse anticipate the patient to demonstrate? _____

    _____

    _____

    b. Discuss the diagnostic tests that may be used in the treatment of the patient and their probable results.

    _____

    _____

Activity 2

37. A patient reports to the emergency department complaining of severe flank pain, nausea, and vomiting. The patient reports that the pain starts in the flank area and radiates to the groin and inner thigh. A urinalysis reveals the presence of hematuria. *(471, 472)*

    a. What medical diagnosis can the nurse anticipate?_____

    _____

   b. Discuss both the conservative and invasive techniques that may be used in the management of this condition.

   _____

   _____

   c. After successful treatment, the nurse is preparing the patient for discharge. Discuss long-term preventive management options. Include diet and medications.

   _____

   _____

Activity 3

38. A 53-year-old man was in a motor vehicle accident 4 days ago. He sustained serious trauma with hypo-volemia that was treated in the emergency department. He has been diagnosed with acute renal failure and is currently in the oliguric phase. *(485, 486)*

   a. What potential clinical manifestations should the nurse be aware of when completing the nursing assessment?

   _____

   _____

   b. Discuss the three phases of acute renal failure. _____

   _____

   _____

   _____

   c. The patient's wife asks if she can bring him a hamburger and fries from a local fast-food restaurant. How will the nurse respond?

   _____

   _____

Activity 4

39. A 22-year-old woman seeks care at the doctor's office complaining of burning with urination, perineal pain, and blood-tinged urine. She is diagnosed with a urinary tract infection. *(464, 465)*

   a. Why are women more prone to urinary tract infections compared to men? _____

   _____

   b. What other signs and symptoms may be present?_____

   _____

   _____

c. What medical treatments can be anticipated in the management of this patient? _____

_____

_____

d. What self-care measures should the nurse suggest to the patient to prevent urinary tract infections?

_____

_____

_____

Care of the Patient with an Endocrine Disorder

chapter

11

Answer Key: Textbook page references are provided as a guide for answering these questions. A complete Answer Key is provided in your Additional Learning Resources on Evolve.

MATCHING

Directions: Match the hormone produced by the gland to the action on the target organ. Indicate your answer in the space provided.

Hormone (Endocrine Gland)

b 1. oxytocin (posterior pituitary) *(500)*

a 2. antidiuretic (posterior pituitary) *(500)*

d 3. thyroxine (thyroid) *(502)*

c 4. calcitonin (thyroid) *(502)*

g 5. parathormone (parathyroid) *(502)*

h 6. mineralocorticoids (adrenal cortex) *(502)*

e 7. glucocorticoids (adrenal cortex) *(502)*

f 8. epinephrine (adrenal medulla) *(503)*

k 9. norepinephrine (adrenal medulla) *(504)*

i 10. insulin (pancreas) *(503)*

l 11. glucagons (pancreas) *(503)*

j 12. melatonin (pineal) *(503)*

Action on Target Organ

a. Causes the kidneys to conserve water by decreasing the amount of urine produced

b. Promotes the release of milk and stimulates uterine contractions during labor

c. Decreases blood calcium levels by causing calcium to be stored in the bones

d. Growth and development; metabolism

e. Involved in glucose metabolism; provides extra reserve energy in times of stress; exhibits antiinflammatory properties

f. Causes the heart rate and blood pressure to increase

g. Increases the concentration of calcium in the blood and regulates phosphorus in the blood

h. Water and electrolyte balance; indirectly manages blood pressure

i. Secreted in response to decreased levels of glucose in the blood

j. Inhibits reproductive activities by inhibiting the gonadotropic hormones

k. Combines with epinephrine to produce "fight-or-flight" response

l. Secreted in response to increased levels of glucose in the blood

FIGURE LABELING

13. Directions: Label the figure below by indicating the position of the glands of the body. *(500)*

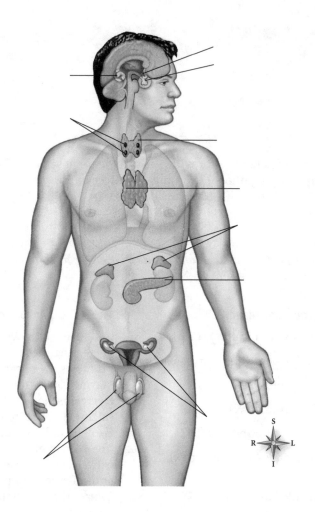

FILL-IN-THE-BLANK SENTENCES

Directions: Complete each sentence by filling in the blank with the correct word or phrase.

14. Diabetes insipidus is a metabolic disorder of the posterior pituitary in which _____ADH_____ is deficient. *(504)*

15. In nondiabetic patients, the beta cells are stimulated by increased blood glucose levels; insulin secretion reaches peak levels about __30__ minutes after meals and returns to normal in __2-3__ hours. *(526)*

16. In type 2 diabetes, the main problem is an abnormal resistance to _____Insulin_____ action. *(526)*

17. Patients should be educated that complications from diabetes can be greatly decreased by proper maintenance of the blood glucose levels of __60-99__ and by appropriate HbA$_{1c}$ levels of less than __5-6__. *(527)*

18. A patient with type 2 diabetes mellitus often has a history of _____obesity_____, _____HTN_____, _____dyslipidemia_____, hypercholesterolemia, and cardiovascular risk (MI, stroke) before the disease is diagnosed. *(527)*

19. _____ causes more cases of blindness in the United States than any other disease. *(538)*

20. Approximately __45%__ of diabetic patients have to undergo either peritoneal dialysis or hemodialysis as a result of vascular changes that affect the kidney. *(539)*

TABLE ACTIVITY

21. Directions: Complete the table below with the correct information about different types of insulin. *(532)*

Type of Insulin	Injection Time (Before Meal)	Risk Time for Hypoglycemic Reaction	Peak Action	Duration
Lispro (Humalog)	5-15 min	No meal within 30 min		
Regular Humulin R Novolin R		Delayed meal or 3-4 hr after injection		2-4 hr
NPH/Regular Mix 70/30 Humulin Mix 70/30	30-60 min		30-60 min	6-12 hr
Lente		3-6 hr after injection		6-12 hr
Glargine (Lantus)	Usually take at 9 PM, once daily		1-2 hr	
Ultralente		6 hr after injection	4-6 hr	

MULTIPLE CHOICE

Directions: Select the best answer(s) for each of the following questions.

22. The nurse is talking to a 31-year-old woman who was recently diagnosed with acromegaly. The woman says, "My career is over. I'll become so hideous, I'm sure that I'll get fired." What is the most therapeutic response? *(504)*
    1. "You have talents and abilities; surely those qualities will be considered."
    2. "Why don't you wait and cross that bridge when you come to it?"
    3. "You are thinking about how your life and career might change."
    4. "Let's talk about what you could do to enhance your appearance."

23. The school nurse is taking the height and weight measurements of all of the children at the beginning of the school year. Measurement for one of the students shows a deviation over two percentile levels from the median. What should the nurse do? *(506)*
    1. Call the parents and ask about the child's birth weight and growth patterns.
    2. Contact the parents and suggest they take the child to the health care provider.
    3. Recheck the child's height and weight once a month for the next several months.
    4. Track the child's growth over time and compare findings to siblings and classmates.

24. Which nursing interventions should be employed for a patient with diabetes insipidus? (Select all that apply.) *(508)*
    1. Assessment of skin turgor
    2. Daily weight measurement
    3. Fluid restriction
    4. Monitor intake and output
    5. Frequent ambulation

25. Which patient has the greatest risk for developing syndrome of inappropriate antidiuretic hormone (SIADH)? *(509)*
    1. Has malignant cancer
    2. Has dormant tuberculosis
    3. Suffered head trauma
    4. Received opiate medication

26. The nurse is caring for a patient who is diagnosed with SIADH. Which assessment finding indicates that the disorder has progressed to neurologic involvement? *(509)*
    1. An increased urge to drink fluids
    2. A decrease in serum sodium
    3. Progression to shock symptoms
    4. A change in mental status

27. For the patient with SIADH, the health care provider orders fluid restriction. Which finding best indicates that the therapy is working? *(509)*
    1. Patient reports that he feels better.
    2. Vital signs are at patient's baseline.
    3. Serum sodium is gradually increased.
    4. Diuretics are gradually discontinued.

28. The nurse is caring for a patient who had a thyroidectomy. Which routine postoperative intervention would the nurse clarify with the health care provider? *(513)*
    1. Inspect dressing for bleeding and drainage.
    2. Give clear liquids; progress to soft diet.
    3. Encourage coughing and deep-breathing.
    4. Observe surgical site for signs of infection.

29. The patient tells the nurse that the health care provider wants to test her for Graves' disease. What symptoms is the patient most likely to exhibit? *(511)*
    1. Weight loss, increased appetite, and nervousness
    2. Intolerance to cold, constipation, and lethargy
    3. Skeletal pain, pain on weight-bearing, and paranoia
    4. Polyphagia, polydipsia, and polyuria

30. The nurse is reviewing the patient's medication orders and sees that the patient is prescribed levothyroxine (Synthroid). Which laboratory result will indicate efficacy of therapy? *(515)*
    1. Blood glucose less than 250 mg/dL
    2. Normalization of urine specific gravity
    3. Gradual improvement of serum sodium level
    4. Normalization of thyroid-stimulating hormone level

31. The nurse is caring for a patient who had a thyroidectomy 6 hours ago. The patient now exhibits extreme anxiety and irritability with a severe elevation in pulse, blood pressure, and temperature. The nurse would initiate emergency measures for which postoperative complication? *(513)*
    1. Hypovolemic shock
    2. Thyroid crisis
    3. Airway obstruction
    4. Septic shock

32. The nurse reads in the patient's chart that a firm, fixed, small, rounded, painless nodule was felt during palpation of the thyroid gland. The nurse prepares to support the patient when the health care provider informs about the need for diagnostic testing for: *(517)*
    1. myxedema.
    2. colloid goiter.
    3. thyroid cancer.
    4. cretinism.

33. The nurse is caring for a patient who has a pathologic fracture secondary to hyperparathyroidism. Which food needs to be taken off the patient's breakfast tray? *(519)*
    1. Glass of whole milk
    2. White toast with jam
    3. Sugared cereal flakes
    4. Fried egg with bacon

34. Why is the diuretic medication furosemide (Lasix) prescribed for a patient with hyperparathyroidism? *(519)*
    1. Preserve existing kidney function
    2. Decrease fluid retention and edema
    3. Encourage the elimination of serum calcium
    4. Decrease blood pressure

35. The LPN is assisting an RN with a patient who needs emergency administration of calcium gluconate for hypoparathyroid tetany. The RN is preparing the medication. What task should the LPN/LVN perform under the supervision of the RN? *(520)*
    1. Assess the patient for medication allergies.
    2. Place the patient on electrocardiographic monitoring.
    3. Assess the patency of the intravenous access.
    4. Verify the order for calcium gluconate.

36. For patients who have hypoparathyroidism, why is it important for the nurse to encourage foods such as soy milk, white rice, jam, honey, lemon-lime soda, cucumbers, lettuce, peppers, tomatoes, and non-organ meats? *(520)*
    1. These foods supply extra calcium, which is needed to treat hypocalcemia.
    2. These foods are low in phosphorus, and serum phosphorus is elevated.
    3. These foods supply vitamin D, which improves the absorption of calcium.
    4. These foods are low in fat and will not be metabolized into ketones.

37. Urine excreted by a patient with diabetes insipidus will exhibit which characteristics? *(507)*
    1. Dilute, with a specific gravity of 1.005–1.030 g/mL
    2. Dilute, with a specific gravity of 1.001–1.005 g/mL
    3. Concentrated, with a specific gravity of 1.005–1.030 g/mL
    4. Concentrated, with a specific gravity of 1.001–1.005 g/mL

38. A patient asks what causes his unsightly goiter. Based on knowledge of pathophysiology, what does the nurse tells the patient? *(516)*
    1. The growth is harmless, like a fluid-filled cyst that can be drained.
    2. There is fluid retention in the face and neck because of a blockage.
    3. The gland usually enlarges because of lack of iodine in the diet.
    4. The surrounding tissue becomes inflamed and swollen because of infection.

39. Cortisol is responsible for what bodily function? *(502)*
    1. Regulates sodium levels
    2. Regulates potassium levels
    3. Provides energy during stress
    4. Responds to decreased glucose levels

40. What type of insulin administration is indicated in the management of hyperglycemia related to diabetic ketoacidosis? *(541)*
    1. Lente insulin given subcutaneously
    2. Ultralente insulin given subcutaneously
    3. NPH 70/30 given intravenously
    4. Regular insulin given intravenously

41. A patient is diagnosed with corticosteroid-induced Cushing's syndrome. Which statement by the patient indicates a need for additional patient teaching? *(522)*
    1. "I would like to try a dose reduction."
    2. "I am going to stop taking the medication."
    3. "I prefer trying a gradual discontinuation."
    4. "I am changing to the alternate-day regimen."

42. The patient with Cushing's syndrome has high risk for impaired skin integrity. What instructions will the nurse give to the UAP to prevent skin impairment? *(522)*
    1. Handle very gently to prevent bruising and ecchymosis.
    2. Assess for signs of erythema, edema, or infection.
    3. Frequently wash the skin to prevent irritation.
    4. Assist females to remove extra hair with a safety razor.

43. The nurse is caring for a patient who is admitted with Addison's disease. During the AM assessment, the nurse notes very high temperature and orthostatic hypotension. Laboratory results show hyponatremia and hyperkalemia. How does the nurse interpret these findings? *(523)*
    1. These are expected findings for this disorder; continue routine assessment.
    2. The frequency of assessment should be increased; reassess status every 1-2 hours.
    3. These are signs of impending addisonian crisis; notify the health care provider.
    4. These should be documented as abnormal findings; compare data for trends.

44. The principal manifestation of pheochromocytoma is severe hypertension. What other symptoms are likely to accompany the excessive secretion of catecholamines (i.e., epinephrine and norepinephrine)? *(525)*
    1. Lethargy, constipation, and depression
    2. Tachycardia, diaphoresis, and anxiety
    3. Kussmaul's respiration, hypotension, and drowsiness
    4. Excessive thirst, increased urine output, and lethargy

45. Which diagnostic test is the best for monitoring long-term compliance for patients with diabetes mellitus? *(529)*
    1. Fasting blood glucose (FBG)
    2. Postprandial (after a meal) blood glucose (PPBG)
    3. Patient self-monitoring of blood glucose (SMBG)
    4. Glycosylated hemoglobin (HbA$_{1c}$)

46. Which patient needs to test the urine for ketones as part of their self-care management? *(527)*
    1. Gestational diabetic who has started insulin
    2. Type 2 diabetic who is preparing to exercise
    3. Type 1 diabetic who has a febrile infection
    4. An older diabetic who cannot perform SMBG

47. The pharmacy delivers a bag of insulin to be delivered as a piggyback infusion. The label says that 100 units of regular insulin is mixed in 500 mL of normal saline. How many mL would be required to deliver 3 units per hour? _____ *(541)*

48. A nurse hears in shift report that a diabetic patient has been NPO since midnight for a surgical procedure that should happen this morning. On assessment, the patient is irritable, and his skin is cool and clammy. His blood glucose is 45 mg/dL. What should the nurse do first? *(540)*
    1. Give the patient some juice and a peanut butter sandwich.
    2. Administer 50% glucose per emergency protocol.
    3. Call the operating room and cancel the procedure.
    4. Call the health care provider and inform about findings.

CRITICAL THINKING ACTIVITIES

Activity 1

49. A 19-year-old woman seeks care because of excessive thirst, hunger, and fatigue. She reports she has not been able to sleep all night for the past few weeks because of needing to go to the bathroom. *(528, 536, 538)*

    a. Based on the nurse's knowledge, what medical diagnosis is anticipated? _____

    _____

    b. What other clinical manifestations may occur in this patient? _____

    _____

    _____

    _____

    _____

c. Describe what the nurse will teach the patient about administering insulin. _____

_____

_____

_____

_____

d. Upon realizing this condition is not curable, the patient asks what acute and long-term complications are associated with diabetes. How will the nurse respond to this inquiry?

_____

_____

_____

_____

Activity 2

50. The parents of a 6-year-old boy report to the health care provider with concerns about their son's height. They report that he is the smallest child in the school. The parents are of normal stature. Assessment reveals that the child is indeed significantly small for his age. *(507)*

a. What diagnostic tests can be anticipated? _____

_____

_____

b. What other clinical manifestations may be exhibited by a child with dwarfism? _____

_____

_____

c. Another question voiced by the parents concern future implications for their child. How will the nurse respond?

_____

_____

_____

d. What medical treatment will be prescribed for this patient? _____

_____

_____

Activity 3

51. Discuss considerations for older adults related to endocrine disorders. *(538)* _____

_____

_____

_____

_____

Activity 4

52. Why should patients with endocrine disorders be advised to wear medical alert jewelry? *(511, 518, 538)*

_____

_____

_____

_____

Care of the Patient with a Reproductive Disorder

Answer Key: Textbook page references are provided as a guide for answering these questions. A complete Answer Key is provided in your Additional Learning Resources on Evolve.

FIGURE LABELING

1. Directions: Label the parts of the female reproductive organs. *(552)*

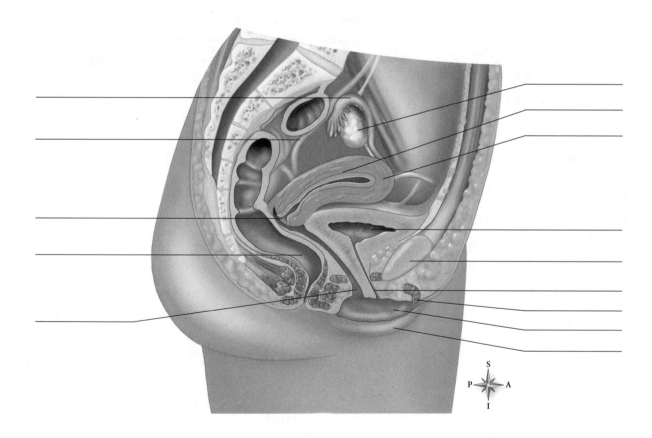

MATCHING

Directions: Match the birth control method with the description. Indicate your answers in the spaces provided. (613-615)

		Method		**Description**

		Method		**Description**
_____	2.	combination pill	a.	Take two within 72 hours of coitus; repeat if vomiting occurs; take second dose 12 hours later
_____	3.	morning-after pill	b.	Consists of a thin flexible rod, which is inserted subdermally
_____	4.	progestin-only pill		
_____	5.	medroxyprogesterone (Depo-Provera)	c.	Rubber thimble-shaped shield covering cervix, held in place by suction
_____	6.	Implanon	d.	Device inserted into uterus; flexible object made of plastic or copper wire
_____	7.	diaphragm	e.	No pill-free days
_____	8.	cervical cap	f.	Double-ring system fitted into vagina up to 8 hours before intercourse
_____	9.	male condom	g.	Contains both estrogen and progesterone
_____	10.	female condom	h.	Only drug given by injection every 3 months
_____	11.	intrauterine device	i.	Dome-shaped latex cap with flexible metal ring
_____	12.	rhythm method	j.	Thin rubber sheath fitting over erect penis
_____	13.	tubal sterilization	k.	Bilateral surgical ligation and resection of ductus deferens
_____	14.	hysterectomy	l.	Crushing, ligating, clipping, or plugging of fallopian tubes
_____	15.	vasectomy	m.	Requires periodic abstinence during fertile portion of menstrual cycle
			n.	Surgical removal of uterus; 100% effective

FILL-IN-THE-BLANK SENTENCES

Directions: Complete each sentence by filling in the blank with the correct word or phrase.

16. Prostate enlargement is increasingly common with each decade after _____ years of age. *(555)*

17. By _____ years of age, children are aware that they will remain boys or girls and that no outward change in their appearance will alter this. *(555)*

18. It is believed that the average breast tumor is present for _____ years before it is palpable. *(560)*

19. All pregnancy tests, regardless of method, are based on detection of _____, which is secreted in the urine after the fertilization of the ovum. *(561)*

20. The appearance of the male climacteric phase is gradual and occurs between _____ and _____ years of age. *(570)*

TRUE OR FALSE

Directions: Write T for true or F for false in the blanks provided.

_____   21.   The hymen can only be ruptured during sexual intercourse. *(553)*

_____ 22. In giving patients information about sexuality, the implication is that the nurse agrees with specific beliefs. *(556)*

_____ 23. CA-125 can detect primary ovarian cancer. *(561)*

_____ 24. Delaying childbearing by women with endometriosis is not recommended as worsening of the condition may result in a loss of fertility. *(579)*

SHORT ANSWER

Directions: Using your own words, answer each question in the space provided.

25. Identify three functions of the organs of the male reproductive system. *(550)*

a. _____

b. _____

c. _____

26. Nurses may intervene in sexual problems among patient populations through what four strategies? *(557)*

a. _____

b. _____

c. _____

d. _____

27. What are the most common disturbances related to menstruation? *(562)*

a. _____

b. _____

c. _____

d. _____

e. _____

28. What are the major goals of treatment of vaginal infections? *(575)*

a. _____

b. _____

c. _____

d. _____

29. What are the four main factors that contribute to STIs being among the world's most common communicable diseases? *(606)*

a. _____

b. _____

c. _____

d. _____

FIGURE LABELING

30. Directions: Label the lymph nodes of the axilla. *(591)*

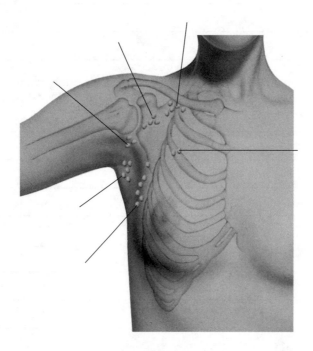

MULTIPLE CHOICE

Directions: Select the best answer(s) for each of the following questions.

31. Which illnesses can result in actual inabilities to function sexually? (Select all that apply.) *(557)*
    1. Diabetes mellitus
    2. End-stage renal disease
    3. Primary syphilis
    4. Hypertension
    5. Spinal cord injuries

32. Which woman needs to be advised to have an annual Pap smear? *(558)*
    1. A 17-year-old who has been sexually active since age 14
    2. A 19-year-old who has never been sexually active
    3. A 31-year-old who had three normal consecutive Pap smears
    4. A 25-year-old who had a hysterectomy for traumatic injury

33. In caring for men who have had diagnostic testing of the reproductive system, the nurse would provide the comfort measures of scrotal support and an ice application for which diagnostic test? *(561)*
    1. Semen analysis
    2. Prostatic smear
    3. Testicular biopsy
    4. Prostate-specific antigen

34. Following a cystoscopy, which finding would be considered normal? *(561)*
    1. Elevated temperature
    2. Decreased urinary output
    3. Pink-tinged urine
    4. Low-back pain

35. For which condition is the nurse most likely to use a heat application as a comfort measure? *(564)*
    1. Amenorrhea
    2. Dysmenorrhea
    3. Menorrhagia
    4. Metrorrhagia

36. The nurse is interviewing a patient who reports that her menstrual periods seem heavier than usual. Which question(s) would the nurse ask? (Select all that apply.) *(566)*
    1. "How many days have you had menstrual flow?"
    2. "How many days would your period typically last?"
    3. "How many pads or tampons are you saturating per day?"
    4. "How frequently would you normally change a pad/tampon?"
    5. "Do you take aspirin or other anticoagulant medications?"
    6. "Have you recently started a rigorous exercise program?"

37. Which disorder is most likely to be treated with an antidepressant medication? *(567)*
    1. Premenstrual dysphoric disorder
    2. Premenstrual syndrome
    3. Pelvic inflammatory disease
    4. Polycystic ovarian syndrome

38. A 55-year-old woman reports that she went through menopause 3 years ago, but has started to have menstrual flow again and she wonders if she should start using birth control again. What should the nurse say? *(586)*
    1. "Resuming birth control is a good idea if you don't want to get pregnant."
    2. "Pregnancy is probably not likely since you went through menopause three years ago."
    3. "Vaginal bleeding after menopause is not expected. See your health care provider."
    4. "Does your current flow look like it did before you went through menopause?"

39. What is the physiologic rationale that supports use of calcium and vitamin D supplements for postmenopausal women? *(569)*
    1. These supplements are an alternative to hormone replacement therapy to relieve hot flashes.
    2. Decreased bone density occurs with menopause; calcium and vitamin D support bone health.
    3. Calcium and vitamin D mimic estrogen and progesterone in their structure and function in the body.
    4. Postmenopausal women are more likely to decrease active exercises that contribute to bone health.

40. For most menopausal women, which symptom/condition could be relieved by the use of a water-soluble lubricant, such as KY? *(570)*
    1. Pruritus
    2. Phimosis
    3. Dyspareunia
    4. Procidentia

41. The woman is undergoing a tubal insufflation test. Which outcome suggests that the fallopian tubes are blocked? *(561)*
    1. No pain or other symptoms are experienced during the test.
    2. The patient experiences shoulder pain during the test.
    3. A high-pitched bubbling is auscultated over the abdomen.
    4. A radiographic film shows free gas under the diaphragm.

42. A 57-year-old male patient confides in the nurse that he doesn't feel as productive or sexually powerful as he used to. What should the nurse say first? *(571)*
    1. "I understand how you feel; aging makes us feel like time is slipping away."
    2. "You'll be okay. Look at all the things you have accomplished so far."
    3. "What factors are contributing to the changes that you see in yourself?"
    4. "Let's talk about ways that you can cope with your loss of sexual power."

43. The nurse is reviewing the medication lists for several patients. Which combination of medications must be immediately brought to the attention of the health care provider? *(572)*
    1. Sildenafil citrate (Viagra) and nitrates (nitroglycerin tablets)
    2. Vitamin B$_6$ supplement and ibuprofen (Motrin)
    3. Cefoxitin (Mefoxin) and steroids (Prednisone)
    4. Danazol (Danocrine) and vitamin E supplement

44. The nurse places the patient with pelvic inflammatory disease in a Fowler's position. What is the rationale for using this position for this patient? *(576)*
    1. Facilitate respiratory effort
    2. Prevent aspiration
    3. Facilitate vaginal drainage
    4. Decrease strain on the abdomen

45. What is an early manifestation of toxic shock syndrome? *(577)*
    1. Decreased urine output
    2. Flulike symptoms
    3. Desquamation of palms
    4. Hypotension

46. What advice does the nurse give about tampon use in order to prevent toxic shock syndrome? *(577)*
    1. Use an applicator to insert super-absorbent tampons.
    2. Wash hands thoroughly after inserting a tampon.
    3. Tampons should be changed every 8 hours.
    4. Alternate the use of tampons with use of pads.

47. Radiation has been scheduled for a patient diagnosed with breast cancer. When developing the plan of care, when should the nurse anticipate radiation will take place? *(595)*
    1. Radiation will begin within 72 hours after surgery.
    2. Radiation will begin within 1 week after surgery.
    3. Radiation will begin 2 to 3 weeks after surgery.
    4. Radiation will begin 4 to 6 weeks after surgery.

48. An advantage of brachytherapy over traditional radiation therapy is that brachytherapy: *(595)*
    1. is more cost-effective.
    2. will take less time to complete.
    3. is associated with fewer side effects.
    4. uses a lower dosage of radiation.

49. Anemia is a side effect associated with chemotherapy. Which medications may be ordered to manage this complication? *(595)*
    1. Epoetin alfa (Procrit)
    2. Prochlorperazine (Compazine)
    3. Granisetron (Kytril)
    4. Ondansetron (Zofran)

50. Tamoxifen has been ordered to manage a patient diagnosed with breast cancer. Which characteristics are associated with tamoxifen? (Select all that apply.) *(595)*
    1. Inhibits the growth-stimulating effects of estrogen
    2. Hormonal agent of choice for postmenopausal women
    3. Used to manage recurrent breast cancer
    4. Used to prevent breast cancer in high-risk individuals
    5. Used for women desiring continued fertility

51. An autologous bone marrow transplant is planned for a patient with breast cancer. Which statement is correct? *(596)*
    1. Radiation is administered before the transplant to reduce the cancerous growth.
    2. Patient will donate bone marrow, from which stem cells will be harvested.
    3. Chemotherapy administration reduces success for the bone marrow transplant.
    4. Plasmapheresis is performed on the donor stem cells before transplantation.

52. A 22-year-old woman who has a history of cervical dysplasia is scheduled for a conization procedure to remove a small eroded area on her cervix. What nursing care is appropriate for this procedure? *(558)*
    1. Assess for allergies to seafood or iodine.
    2. Monitor for bleeding after the procedure.
    3. Encourage fluids prior to the procedure.
    4. Remind to refrain from using deodorants.

53. When teaching a patient about the rationale for prescribing oral contraceptives to treat dysmenorrhea, the nurse's statement is based on the understanding that oral contraceptives will: *(564)*
    1. suppress ovulation by increasing prostaglandin levels.
    2. suppress ovulation by increasing estrogen levels.
    3. suppress ovulation by inhibiting prostaglandin levels.
    4. promote ovulation by increasing estrogen levels.

54. What is the treatment of choice for primary syphilis? *(608)*
    1. Penicillin
    2. Acyclovir
    3. Valtrex
    4. Tetracycline

55. A 22-year-old man comes to the clinic with complaints of urethritis, dysuria, and purulent penile discharge. What medical diagnosis should be anticipated? *(609)*
    1. Genital herpes
    2. Syphilis
    3. Chlamydia
    4. Gonorrhea

56. A patient who has a pessary reports foul-smelling discharge, vaginal irritation, and difficulty with sexual intercourse. Which question should the nurse ask? *(581)*
    1. Have you been using vaginal douching?
    2. Are you having burning with urination?
    3. How long has it been since it was cleaned?
    4. Do you use spermicidals for birth control?

CRITICAL THINKING ACTIVITIES

Activity 1

57. A 20-year-old patient reports to the family planning clinic for painful, erythematous vesicles on her genitals. She is scared and voices many questions and concerns about her condition. *(606, 607)*

    a. Based on the nurse's knowledge, what is anticipated to be her medical diagnosis? _____

    _____

    b. After being advised of her condition, the patient becomes tearful and asks what will be done to cure her. How should the nurse respond to her question?

    _____

    _____

    _____

    _____

    c. What treatment options and interventions are available to the patient? _____

    _____

    _____

    _____

    d. What should be included in her patient education? _____

_____

_____

_____

_____

Activity 2

58. The nurse is preparing to discuss menstruation with a group of preteen girls. The nurse will include the following teaching points. *(562)*

    a. At what age do girls typically begin menstruation? _____

    b. Approximately how much blood is lost during the average menstrual period?_____

    c. List the hormones involved in the menstrual cycle._____

_____

    d. What will the nurse tell the girls about personal hygiene? _____

_____

_____

_____

Activity 3

59. The nurse is originally from a very small farming town in the western United States, but after graduating, she decides to work in an urban clinic that serves an inner-city community in a very large city in the eastern part of the United States. *(606)*

    a. What are the risk factors for the clinic population that are likely to contribute to reproductive disorders?

_____

_____

_____

_____

    b. What can the nurse do to prepare herself to help patients that may have gender identity beliefs or sexual practices that are different from her own?

_____

_____

_____

_____

Activity 4

60. Discuss the emotional impact for a couple who is undergoing diagnostic testing for infertility. *(574)*

_____

_____

_____

_____

_____

_____

_____

_____

Care of the Patient with a Visual or Auditory Disorder

Answer Key: Textbook page references are provided as a guide for answering these questions. A complete Answer Key is provided in your Additional Learning Resources on Evolve.

FIGURE LABELING

1. Directions: Label the anatomy of the eye. *(622)*

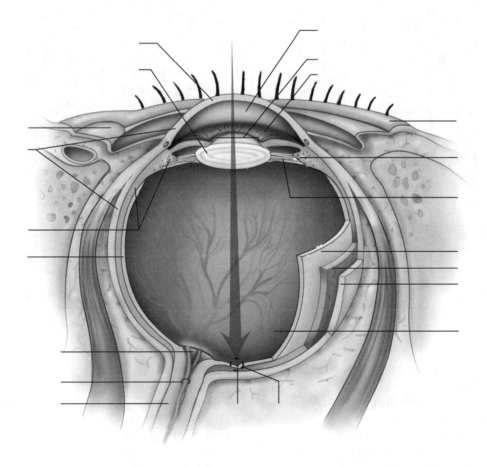

CROSSWORD PUZZLE

2. Use the clues to complete the crossword puzzle.

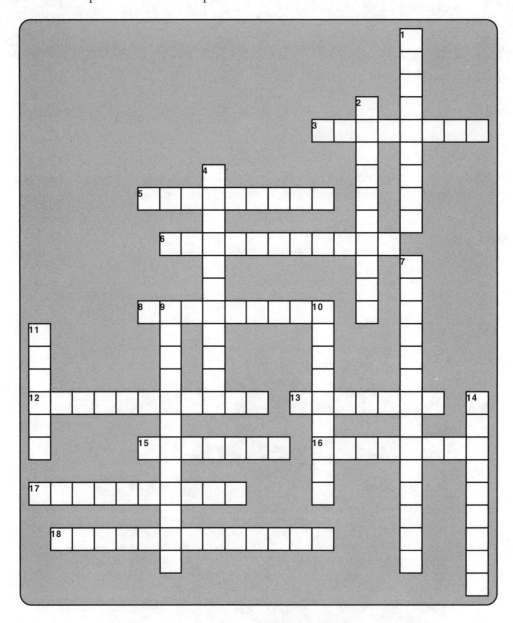

Across

3. Crystalline opacity or clouding of the lens *(634)*
5. Inflammation of the cornea *(632)*
6. Defect in curvature of eyeball surface *(628)*
8. Infection of eyelid margin *(630)*
12. A hearing deficit secondary to aging *(665)*
13. Agents that cause the pupil to constrict *(643)*
15. Sensation of moving or spinning *(652)*
16. Ringing or tinkling sounds in the ear *(656)*
17. A type of refractory error *(625)*
18. Inflammation of the labyrinthine canals of the inner ear *(658)*

Down

1. Farsightedness *(628)*
2. Cross-eyed *(628)*
4. Infection of one of the mastoid bones *(658)*
7. Pinkeye *(631)*
9. Chronic progressive deafness caused by the formation of spongy bone *(660)*
10. Dilating drops *(625)*
11. Nearsightedness *(628)*
14. Involuntary, rhythmic movements of the eyes *(652)*

TRUE OR FALSE

Directions: Write T for true or F for false in the blanks provided.

_____ 3. Most cataracts are caused by chronic eye infections. *(634)*

_____ 4. The incidence of diabetic retinopathy greatly increases in relation to how long the patient has diabetes mellitus and how well their blood glucose levels are controlled. *(636)*

_____ 5. Central vision damaged by macular degeneration can be restored by photocoagulation. *(639)*

_____ 6. There is a direct relationship between vascular hypertension and ocular hypertension. *(644)*

_____ 7. The deaf community believes that life without hearing is healthy and functional and that deafness is not a disease that needs to be cured. *(665)*

FILL-IN-THE-BLANK SENTENCES

Directions: Complete each sentence by filling in the blank with the correct word or phrase.

8. The normal visual field range is _____ degrees. *(626)*

9. A patient with glaucoma tests above the normal range of _____ mm Hg. *(642)*

10. Primary open-angle glaucoma is medically treated by the use of beta blockers, _____, and carbonic anhydrase inhibitors. *(643)*

11. The four taste sensations are _____, _____, _____, and _____. *(664)*

SHORT ANSWER

Directions: Using your own words, answer each question in the space provided.

12. What four basic processes are necessary to form an image? *(624)*

   a. _____

   b. _____

   c. _____

   d. _____

13. Define the following types of blindness. *(626)*

   a. Total blindness: _____

   b. Functional blindness: _____

   c. Legal blindness: _____

14. What group of disorders characterizes glaucoma? *(641)*

   a. _____

   b. _____

   c. _____

15. Briefly define the six types of hearing loss. *(653)*

a. _____

b. _____

c. _____

d. _____

e. _____

f. _____

FIGURE LABELING

16. Directions: Label the anatomy of the external, middle, and inner ear. *(649)*

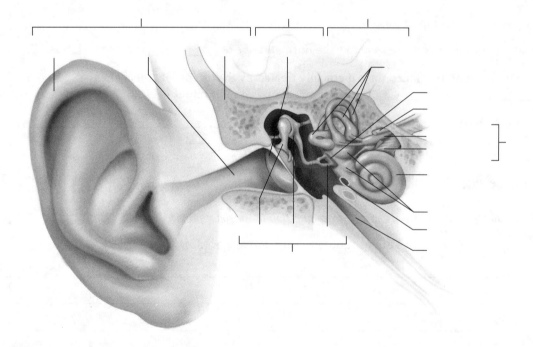

MULTIPLE CHOICE

Directions: select the best answer(s) for each of the following questions.

17. The patient shows loss and deterioration in the automated perimetry test. Which activity is the patient most likely to have difficulty with? *(625)*
    1. Reading a newspaper or book
    2. Driving through the neighborhood
    3. Looking at a laptop computer screen
    4. Going on a moonlight stroll down the street

18. Which diagnostic test requires an assessment of allergies to seafood or iodine? *(625)*
    1. Snellen's test
    2. Slit-lamp examination
    3. Fluorescein angiography
    4. Tonometry

19. The nurse hears in the shift report that the patient has diplopia. Which task will be the most difficult for the patient? *(626)*
    1. Sitting upright in bed
    2. Reading an information brochure
    3. Listening to a radio broadcast
    4. Eating a sandwich with fries

20. The nurse is orienting the patient to the hospital environment. He is just learning to use a cane as an assistive device for partial blindness. Which interventions would the nurse use? (Select all that apply.) *(626)*
    1. Walk silently beside the patient, so that he can hear environmental noises.
    2. Suggest that the cane be used to identify borders or objects in pathways.
    3. Walk behind the patient, so that the pathway is clear for him/her.
    4. Advise to walk slowly, especially since the environment is unfamiliar.
    5. Describe the general layout of the room and the adjacent hallway.

21. For which eye condition are patients most likely to report trying to first self-treat with over-the-counter eyewear? *(629)*
    1. Astigmatism
    2. Strabismus
    3. Myopia
    4. Hyperopia

22. A patient with myopia is thinking about having refractory surgery to correct the problem. What should the patient do prior to the surgery? *(629)*
    1. Arrange to take at least 2 weeks off from work for recuperation.
    2. Stop wearing contact lenses for 1 to 2 weeks before surgical evaluation.
    3. Stop taking any medications for at least 2 days before the surgery.
    4. Use sterile hydrating eyedrops for at least 2 weeks prior to surgery.

23. The nurse's teenage son tells her that his contact lens fell out while he was hanging out in the park with his friends, so he used saliva to clean it off. What should the nurse say? *(630)*
    1. "Did you ask if anybody had contact lens solution or a lens case?"
    2. "You know you are not supposed to do that, don't you?"
    3. "So, what are you planning to do if that happens again?"
    4. "Do you think glasses would be a better option for you?"

24. The nurse has a 10-year-old daughter who wants to invite two friends for a sleepover. Part of the entertainment for the night is to do "glamour makeovers." What should the nurse do? *(646)*
    1. Tell the daughter that sharing eye makeup contributes to eye infections.
    2. Call the other parents and see if the friends currently have eye infections.
    3. Purchase three makeup kits from the drugstore and supervise the activity.
    4. Teach the children how to use a fresh cotton-tip applicator for application.

25. The home health nurse is supervising a parent who is demonstrating care for her child's conjunctivitis. The nurse would intervene if the mother performed which action? *(632)*
    1. Used a clean washcloth to wipe away the secretions
    2. Applied a warm compress with a clean cloth for comfort
    3. Instilled the eyedrops in the lower conjunctival sac
    4. Taped an eyepad loosely over the affected eye

26. For a patient who is diagnosed with keratitis, which common symptom differentiates this disease from other inflammatory eye diseases? *(632)*
    1. Elevated body temperature
    2. Severe eye pain
    3. Presence of halos or flashes
    4. Low white cell count

27. A patient has recently been diagnosed with keratoconjunctivitis sicca and a dry mouth. Which immune disorder is likely to be associated with this diagnosis and symptom? *(633)*
    1. Sjögren's syndrome
    2. Acquired immunodeficiency syndrome
    3. Rheumatoid arthritis
    4. Type 1 diabetes mellitus

28. Patients with Sjögren's syndrome typically report: *(633)*
    1. seeing floaters in the field of vision.
    2. color blindness.
    3. feeling worse in the morning.
    4. feeling that their eyes are gritty.

29. Ectropion is often characterized by: (Select all that apply.) *(634)*
    1. tearing.
    2. redness of sclera.
    3. thick eye discharge.
    4. corneal dryness.
    5. outward turning of eyelid margin.

30. What diagnostic tests are used to confirm the presence of entropion? *(634)*
    1. Amsler's grid
    2. Snellen's examination
    3. Ophthalmologic examination
    4. Pneumatic retinopexy

31. The typical type of visual distortions associated with diabetic retinopathy will include: *(638)*
    1. tunnel vision that worsens in low lighting.
    2. a loss of visual acuity accompanied by "floaters."
    3. a sudden onset of peripheral vision loss and eye discomfort.
    4. reddened eyes accompanied by a yellow discharge.

32. A 65-year-old patient reports to the office complaining of visual deficits, including disturbances in color vision and visual clarity, and a darkened area in the center of vision. What medical diagnosis does the nurse anticipate will be made? *(639)*
    1. Macular degeneration
    2. Glaucoma
    3. Herpetic keratitis
    4. Cataracts

33. Tonometry is used in the diagnosis of what condition? *(642)*
    1. Corneal abrasions
    2. Blepharitis
    3. Glaucoma
    4. Retinal detachment

34. The patient has been diagnosed with a visual disorder. Contact lenses have been prescribed. Which statement indicates the need for further instruction? *(629)*
    1. "Photophobia, dryness, burning, or tearing are expected symptoms."
    2. "I will use proper lens care solutions and a clean lens case."
    3. "I will need to be careful not to mix up my left and right lenses."
    4. "Washing and drying my hands before handling my lenses is essential."

35. Following cataract surgery, which activity is the ophthalmologist most likely to discourage? *(635)*
    1. Going to the movies
    2. Lifting a grandchild
    3. Walking on a sunny day
    4. Sleeping with a spouse

36. Based on research, supplemental zinc, beta-carotene, vitamins C and E, and a diet rich in fruits and dark-green leafy vegetables would be recommended for which eye disorder? *(638)*
    1. Age-related macular degeneration
    2. Senile cataracts
    3. Retinal detachment
    4. Glaucoma

37. A patient reports seeing flashing lights and floaters and a dark area in the outer peripheral vision. What is the most important question to ask for suspicion of retinal detachment? *(640)*
    1. "Are you having severe pain in the affected eye?"
    2. "Is the darkened area getting progressively larger?"
    3. "Do you have type 1 diabetes mellitus?"
    4. "Do you have a family history of eye problems?"

38. The nurse's neighbor is trying to remove an eyelash that has gotten in her eye. The nurse would intervene if the neighbor used which method? *(646)*
    1. Flushed the eye gently with tap water
    2. Tried blinking and crying to stimulate tears
    3. Used a clean cotton-tipped swab to wipe the cornea
    4. Used a sterile pad to wipe the corner of the eye

39. The nurse is on a camping trip and one of the campers gets poked in the eye with a stick. The end of the stick is protruding from the eye. What should the nurse do first? *(646)*
    1. Gently remove the stick and then flush the eye with water.
    2. Cover the eye and stick with a paper cup and secure with tape.
    3. Have the camper sit quietly in the car and drive him to the hospital.
    4. Remain calm and control the bleeding with direct pressure.

40. The health care provider informs the nurse that the patient had an abnormal Romberg test. Which safety precaution will the nurse initiate? *(652)*
    1. Make sure the room has adequate natural lighting.
    2. Do a physical demonstration of how to use the call light.
    3. Announce self to avoid suddenly startling the patient.
    4. Assist the patient to stand and get balance before walking.

41. The nurse's toddler received a prescription for antibiotics to treat acute otitis media. The antibiotics and acetaminophen where given as recommended, but the toddler is still crying with pain. What should the nurse try first? *(656)*
    1. Have the toddler swallow cool fluids.
    2. Place a warm compress over the affected ear.
    3. Use distraction until the acetaminophen works.
    4. Call the provider and ask for a sedative prescription.

42. The nurse is reviewing the patient's medication list and sees the patient takes meclizine (Antivert). What instructions should be given to the UAP? *(657)*
    1. Face the patient directly when speaking to him.
    2. Assist the patient to ambulate because he gets dizzy.
    3. Keep the head of the bed elevated at least 30 degrees.
    4. Assist the patient to clean his eyes with a clean washcloth.

43. Which intervention applies to positioning the patient after a stapedectomy? *(662)*
    1. Keep the operative side facing upward.
    2. Elevate the head of the bed to at least 90 degrees.
    3. Turn, cough, and deep-breathe every 2 hours.
    4. Use a neck brace for the first 2 hours.

CRITICAL THINKING ACTIVITIES

Activity 1

44. An 18-year-old patient has just returned from surgery for the enucleation of his right eye after injuries suffered in an automobile accident. *(647)*

    a. Discuss the nursing interventions that will be required over the next 24 hours._____

    _____

    _____

    _____

    b. What findings are indicative of complications and warrant an immediate report to the health care provider?

    _____

    c. The patient expresses concerns about his appearance. How will the nurse address his concerns?

    _____

    _____

Activity 2

45. A 20-year-old patient reports worsening ear pain. After completing his history, it is determined he recently had an ear infection and he failed to take the full course of prescribed medications. His other signs and symptoms include fever, headache, malaise, and purulent exudates. *(658)*

    a. What should the nurse anticipate the patient's medical diagnosis will be? _____

    _____

    b. How did this condition occur? _____

    _____

    _____

    c. Discuss the treatment and the prognosis of this condition. _____

    _____

    _____

    _____

    _____

Activity 3

46. The patient had a car accident and is returning to the nurse's unit from vitrectomy surgery of the right eye. List the appropriate nursing interventions for this patient. *(649)*

    _____

    _____

    _____

    _____

    _____

    _____

    _____

Activity 4

47. Refer to Box 13-2 on page 651 and identify behaviors that you have noticed for someone you know who may be demonstrating a hearing loss. Has the person you identified admitted that he or she has a hearing loss?

    _____

    _____

    _____

    _____

Activity 5

48. If you were to suddenly lose your vision or hearing, how would the loss affect your current lifestyle and future plans?

_____

_____

_____

_____

_____

_____

_____

_____

Care of the Patient with a Neurologic Disorder

Answer Key: Textbook page references are provided as a guide for answering these questions. A complete Answer Key is provided in your Additional Learning Resources on Evolve.

FIGURE LABELING

1. Directions: Label the parts of the brain on the figure below. *(673)*

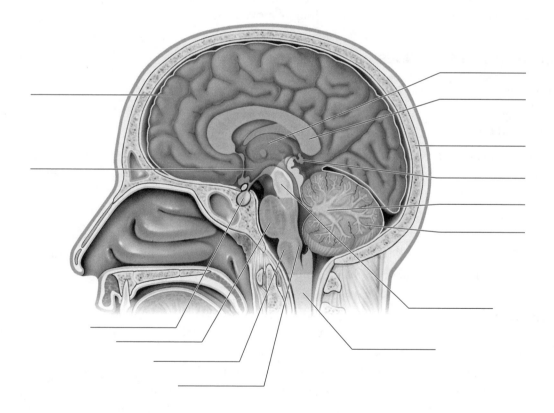

MATCHING

Directions: Match the cranial nerves to their functions. Indicate your answers in the spaces provided. (676)

		Cranial Nerve		**Functions**

_____   2. I—olfactory

_____   3. II—optic

_____   4. III—oculomotor

_____   5. IV—trochlear

_____   6. VI—abducens

_____   7. VII—facial

_____   8. VIII—acoustic (vestibulocochlear)

_____   9. IX—glossopharyngeal

_____   10. X—vagus

_____   11. XI—spinal accessory

_____   12. XII—hypoglossal

a. Eye movements, extraocular muscles, pupillary control (pupillary constriction)
b. Hearing; sense of balance (equilibrium)
c. Down and inward movement of eye
d. Shoulder movements (trapezius muscle) and turning movements of head (sternocleidomastoid muscles)
e. Sense of smell
f. Vision
g. Sense of taste on anterior two-thirds of tongue; contraction of muscles of facial expression
h. Sensations of throat, taste, swallowing movements, gag reflex, taste posterior one-third of tongue, secretion of saliva
i. Lateral movement of eye
j. Sensations of throat, larynx, and thoracic and abdominal organs; swallowing, voice production, slowing of heartbeat, acceleration of peristalsis
k. Tongue movements

FILL-IN-THE-BLANK SENTENCES

Directions: Complete each sentence by filling in the blank with the correct word or phrase.

13. The two main structural divisions of the nervous system are the _____ nervous system and the _____ nervous system. *(733)*

14. The cerebrum is the largest part of the brain and contains five major areas: _____, _____, _____, _____, and _____. *(733)*

15. _____ is a generalized impairment of intellect, awareness, and judgment. *(725)*

16. _____ disease is characterized by abnormal and excessive involuntary writhing and twisting movements of the face, limbs, and body. *(712)*

17. In untreated cases of brain abscess, the mortality rate approaches _____%. *(724)*

TRUE OR FALSE

Directions: Write T for true or F for false in the blanks provided.

_____   18. Pain receptors are not adaptable—they are specific for pain only—and pain impulses continue at the same rate as long as the stimulus is present. *(686)*

_____   19. Amyotrophic lateral sclerosis usually results in death 2 to 6 years after diagnosis. Respiratory tract infection secondary to compromised respiratory function is usually the cause. *(711)*

_____   20. Seventy to eighty percent of people who become infected with the West Nile virus develop encephalitis or meningitis. *(723)*

_____   21. Few patients with advanced HIV disease (AIDS) ever actually develop neurologic symptoms. *(724)*

_____   22. Most elderly people will eventually experience dementia. *(677)*

FIGURE LABELING

23. Directions: In the figure below, identify decorticate and decerebrate responses and the flexion and extension characteristics of the upper and lower extremities. *(689)*

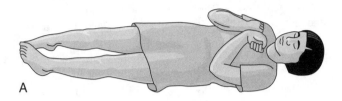

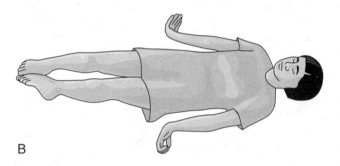

WORD SCRAMBLE

Levels of Consciousness

Directions: Unscramble the letters to reveal the correct spelling of terms related to level of consciousness and then match them to the correct definition or description. (678)

Scrambled Term	Unscrambled Term	Definition or Characteristic
24. treal		
25. orientdisation		
26. porstu		
27. tosecomasemi		
28. esotamoc		

Description
a. Responds to verbal commands with moaning or groaning, if at all; seems unaware of surroundings
b. Is in impaired state of consciousness, characterized by obtundation and stupor, from which a patient can be aroused only by energetic stimulation
c. Unable to respond to painful stimuli; cornea and pupillary reflexes are absent; cannot swallow or cough; is incontinent of urine and feces; electroencephalogram pattern demonstrates decreased or absent neuronal activity
d. Unable to follow simple commands; thinking slowed; inattentive; flat affect
e. Responds appropriately to auditory, tactile, and visual stimuli

MULTIPLE CHOICE

Directions: Select the best answer(s) for each of the following questions.

29. What behavior(s) would be considered normal neurologic changes related to aging? (Select all that apply.) *(677)*
    1. Drives slower to compensate for slowed reaction time
    2. Demonstrates slight tremor while holding teacup when tired
    3. Takes a foreign language class, but can't keep up with classmates
    4. Does needlework, but has more trouble with fine, small stitches
    5. Rearranges items on countertop, but action serves no purpose
    6. Frequently misplaces keys or eyeglasses, but can usually find them

30. The nurse is assessing the "fund of knowledge" component of the patient's awareness. Which question would the nurse use to assess this component? *(678)*
    1. "What month is it? And what day of the week is it today?"
    2. "What did you have for dinner last night?"
    3. "If you had $3.00 and gave me half, what would you have?"
    4. "Who was president before Obama took office?"

31. The nurse is assessing a patient who had a serious head injury. During the assessment, the patient spontaneously opens his eyes; is oriented to person, place, and time; and can follow the nurse's commands. How would the nurse document his Glasgow coma score? *(678)*
    1. GCS within normal limits
    2. GCS insufficient
    3. GCS 3
    4. GCS 15

32. The nurse is using the FOUR Score coma scale to assess a patient who suffered a stroke. Which assessment is an integral part of this scale? *(679)*
    1. Checking the blood pressure and pulse
    2. Checking orientation to person, place, and time
    3. Assessing the respiratory rate and pattern
    4. Evaluating the ability to make good judgments

33. The nurse hears in report that the patient has motor aphasia. Which intervention will the nurse plan to use when communicating with this patient? *(679)*
    1. Talk slower, be patient, and enunciate very clearly.
    2. Face the patient so that he can watch the lips move.
    3. Obtain a set of picture cards and encourage gestures.
    4. Be kind and caring, but limit verbal communication.

34. The nurse is checking the gag reflex prior to giving liquids to a patient who had a bronchoscopy earlier in the day. Which cranial nerve is the nurse testing? *(679, 680)*
    1. Trochlear
    2. Abducens
    3. Trigeminal
    4. Glossopharyngeal

35. The nurse is caring for a patient who has unilateral neglect that includes the nondominant hand. For which task is the patient most likely to require assistance? *(680)*
    1. Putting on her blouse
    2. Brushing her hair
    3. Using the remote control
    4. Writing a letter

36. The patient is scheduled to return from having a lumbar puncture. What instructions will the nurse give to the UAP about the care of this patient? *(681)*
    1. Help the patient ambulate in the halls.
    2. Keep the head of the bed at 30 degrees.
    3. Patient needs to be NPO for several hours.
    4. Report if the patient has numbness or tingling.

37. The nurse is caring for a patient who had cerebral angiography and the vascular system was accessed through the carotid artery. In the immediate postprocedure assessment, what is the priority? *(683)*
    1. Watching for infection at the puncture site
    2. Assessing for reaction to contrast media
    3. Observing for respiratory difficulties
    4. Assessing for nausea and vomiting

38. A 35-year-old man who suffers from tension headaches requests opioid medications for the debilitating pain. Why is the health care provider unlikely to grant the patient's request? *(685)*
    1. Opioids are avoided because of the risk of abuse.
    2. Tension headache pain does not warrant opioid use.
    3. Pain receptor sites will not respond to opioids.
    4. Tension headaches are controlled by reducing stress.

39. Which food may cause or worsen a migraine headache? *(684)*
    1. Italian foods
    2. Apples
    3. Dairy products
    4. Ripened cheese

40. In caring for a patient with a headache, which instruction will the nurse give to the UAP? *(685)*
    1. Assist the patient to turn every 2 hours.
    2. Keep the room quiet and dark.
    3. Refresh warm compress as needed.
    4. Maintain NPO status for nausea.

41. The nurse is reviewing the medication list for a patient who is diabetic and sees that gabapentin (Neurontin) is prescribed. Which pain assessment will the nurse make? *(687)*
    1. Low-back pain with movement
    2. Dull or throbbing headache
    3. Burning or tingling in lower legs
    4. Stiffness in joints in the morning

42. What is an early sign of increased intracranial pressure? *(688)*
    1. Change in level of consciousness
    2. Decreased or abnormal respirations
    3. Increased systolic blood pressure
    4. Increased or widening pulse pressure

43. The nurse is checking the pupils of a patient who sustained a serious head injury. Which pupil response is the most ominous? *(688)*
    1. Pupil reacts, but is sluggish.
    2. Pupil is fixed and dilated.
    3. Pupil is dilated, but will slowly constrict.
    4. Pupil on affected side is larger.

44. Select the measures that may be implemented to reduce venous volume in a patient experiencing increased intracranial pressure. (Select all that apply.) *(690)*
    1. Restrict fluid intake.
    2. Place head in flexed position.
    3. Avoid flexion of the hips.
    4. Administer enemas as needed.
    5. Administer oxygen.

45. The patient has residual hemiplegia following a stroke. Which instructions will the nurse give to the UAP? *(691)*
    1. Assist the patient to ambulate to the bathroom.
    2. Put the unaffected arm through range of motion.
    3. Place in a prone position if the patient can tolerate it.
    4. Use pillows to keep the upper arm in abduction.

46. The nurse hears in report that the 33-year-old patient with multiple sclerosis (MS) is withdrawn, depressed, and emotionally labile. The nurse knows that emotional changes are part of the disease. What other aspect(s) of the disease is/are likely to be contributing to the patient's emotional state? (Select all that apply.) *(699, 700)*
    1. Exacerbations and remissions are continuous; deterioration progresses.
    2. The symptoms are vague, insidious, and widely distributed.
    3. No specific treatments exist, although many treatments have been tried.
    4. Multiple body systems are affected and function is lost in every area.
    5. If cured in the early stages, patient can maintain independence and self-care.

47. A resident with Parkinson's disease lives at a long-term care facility. The patient has a flat facial expression, hand tremors, and bradykinesia. Which instruction will the nurse give to the UAP to address the bradykinesia? *(703)*
    1. He has a shuffling gait and needs assistance to prevent bumping into objects.
    2. He has trouble bending to tie his shoes because of muscle soreness and aches.
    3. He has trouble eating soup or drinking coffee because of fine hand tremors.
    4. He has resistance to motion, so he may seem stiff when you put on his shirt.

48. What is an early subjective symptom that the patient may report that would be characteristic of myasthenia gravis? *(710)*
    1. Muscle weakness in the extremities
    2. Eyelid drooping and double vision
    3. Trouble swallowing
    4. Weak, nasal-sounding voice

49. What is the single most important modifiable risk factor for stroke? *(712)*
    1. Cigarette smoking
    2. Sedentary lifestyle
    3. Hypertension
    4. Obesity

50. The patient who had a stroke exhibits dysphagia. Which intervention will the nurse use? *(692)*
    1. Mix solid and liquid foods together to facilitate swallowing.
    2. Assist the patient to drink water after every bite of food.
    3. Offer the patient a drinking straw or a covered plastic cup.
    4. Check mouth on the affected side for accumulation of food.

51. The patient comes to the clinic and is exhibiting stroke symptoms. The health care provider believes that the patient is a possible candidate for thrombolytic therapy. What are the most important actions for the clinic staff to perform? *(716)*
    1. Rapid triage and transport to a stroke center
    2. Draw blood for coagulation tests and establish IV
    3. Obtain a CT or MRI to rule out hemorrhagic stroke
    4. Explain the risks and benefits of therapy to the patient

52. In caring for a patient with trigeminal neuralgia, what instructions would the nurse give to the UAP about assisting with hygiene and meals? *(719)*
    1. Use gentle touch when assisting with shaving.
    2. Encourage the patient to drink cold liquids.
    3. Ask the patient if he prefers to do his own care.
    4. Offer to cut the patient's food into bite-sized pieces.

53. A patient who is diagnosed with Bell's palsy will need to know how to use which device? *(720)*
    1. Eating utensil with a universal cuff
    2. Eyeshield to be applied at night
    3. Footboard for the end of the bed
    4. A volar wrist splint for extension

54. In caring for a patient who is diagnosed with Guillain-Barré syndrome (GBS), what is the priority assessment? *(722)*
    1. Paralysis in the legs
    2. Respiratory function
    3. Change of mental status
    4. Loss of bowel control

55. The nurse is caring for a patient who is diagnosed with bacterial meningitis. For this patient, what is the rationale for keeping the room quiet and dark? *(723)*
    1. Light and noise increase the subjective experience of pain.
    2. Patient needs extra rest and sleep to facilitate recovery.
    3. Any increased sensory stimulation may cause a seizure.
    4. Critically ill patients do better in quiet environments.

56. What is considered a prominent early sign of a brain tumor? *(725)*
    1. Speech impairment
    2. Morning headache
    3. Change in personality
    4. Memory loss

57. A young man who sustained a serious head injury several years ago is a resident in a long-term care facility. After the injury, he demonstrated intermittent poor judgment and occasional physical aggression. Today, he is trying to leave the facility. What should the nurse do first? *(728)*
    1. Speak calmly and redirect him to another activity.
    2. Obtain an order for a PRN antianxiety medication.
    3. Allow him to wander around, but keep an eye on him.
    4. Instruct a UAP to perform one-on-one observation.

58. The UAP tells the nurse that a patient with a spinal cord injury has a systolic blood pressure of 190/100 mm Hg. The nurse observes that the patient is diaphoretic, restless, and has "gooseflesh" and a headache. What should the nurse do first? *(729)*
    1. Recheck the blood pressure.
    2. Check the bladder for distention.
    3. Check the rectum for impaction.
    4. Put the patient in a sitting position.

CRITICAL THINKING ACTIVITIES

Activity 1

59. The school nurse is accompanying a group of children on a field trip. One of children suddenly reports feeling odd and then sits down on the ground. As the nurse eases her to a supine position, the child demonstrates tonic-clonic jerking movements of the body. The nurse notes secretions and drooling from the child's mouth and the lips are slightly cyanotic. The child is unable to respond to her name and her eyes are rolled back and upwards. *(695, 698)*

    a. Describe what the nurse should do. _____

    _____

    _____

    b. What information should the nurse record and report to the health care provider? _____

    _____

    _____

Activity 2

60. A 58-year-old man reports he experienced numbness in his legs, a loss of sensation in his arms, and an inability to speak. Upon questioning, he reported that the entire event lasted only about 15 minutes. *(714)*

    a. What condition/disorder has the patient experienced? _____

    b. Since this event was short in duration, is it of any long-term significance? Why or why not? *(714)*

    _____

    _____

    _____

    c. What is the most frequently prescribed antiplatelet agent for this condition? *(714)*_____

    _____

Activity 3

61. a. It is likely that you know or will know someone who has Alzheimer's disease. What are the warning signs? *(708, 709)*

_____

_____

_____

_____

    b. Discuss the effect that Alzheimer's disease has on family and society. *(708, 709)* _____

_____

_____

_____

_____

    c. What are things you can do and teach your patients to do that will help prevent Alzheimer's disease? *(708, 709)*

_____

_____

_____

_____

Care of the Patient with an Immune Disorder

chapter

15

Answer Key: Textbook page references are provided as a guide for answering these questions. A complete Answer Key is provided in your Additional Learning Resources on Evolve.

FIGURE LABELING

1. Directions: Label the figure below with the correct names of the organs of the immune system. *(739)*

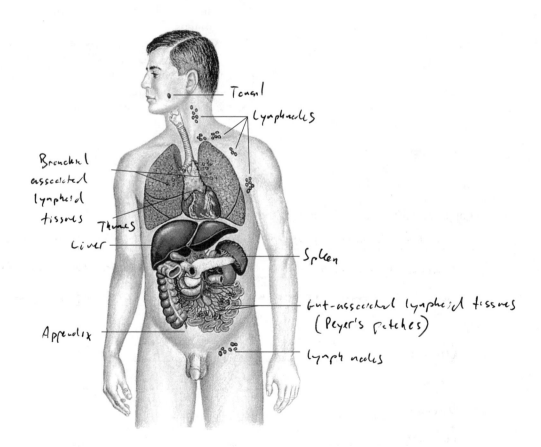

Tonsil

Lymphnodes

Bronchial associated lymphoid tissues

Thymus

Liver

Spleen

Gut-associated lymphoid tissues (Peyer's patches)

Appendix

Lymph nodes

MATCHING

Directions: Match the term related to the immune system with the defining characteristics.

	Term		Defining Characteristics
c	2. autoimmune disorders *(738)*	a.	Provides a specific reaction to each invading antigen and has the unique ability to remember the antigen that caused the attack
d	3. innate system *(738)*	b.	Immune response is too weak or too vigorous and system malfunctions
b	4. immunoincompetence *(737)*	c.	Systemic lupus erythematosus, celiac disease, thyroid disease, inflammatory bowel disease, type I diabetes, multiple sclerosis, myasthenia gravis, psoriasis, rheumatoid arthritis
a	5. adaptive immunity *(739)* – memory – second line of defense		
f	6. allergen *(740)*	d.	Includes intact skin and mucous membranes, cilia, stomach acid, tears, saliva, sebaceous glands, and secretions and flora of the intestines and vagina
e	7. immunization *(740)*	e.	Process by which resistance to an infectious disease is induced or increased
h	8. active immunity *(740)*	f.	Substance that can produce a hypersensitive reaction in the body, but may not be inherently harmful
i	9. cellular immunity *(740)*	g.	Caused by hyperactive responses against environmental antigens
j	10. complement system *(741)*	h.	Antibodies produced by one's own body
g	11. allergies *(738)*	i.	Negative effects include rejection of transplanted tissues, contact hypersensitivity reactions, and certain autoimmune diseases
		j.	Functions in a "step-by-step" series

SHORT ANSWER

Directions: Using your own words, answer each question in the space provided.

12. What are the three main functions of the immune system? *(737)*

    a. Protect body's internal environment against invading microorganisms.

    b. Maintain homeostasis by removing damaged cells from the circulation.

    c. Surveillance network for recognizing against the development and growth of abnormal cells

13. What are the four Rs of the immune response? *(740)*

    a. Recognize

    b. Respond

    c. Remember

    d. Regulate

14. Identify the five factors influencing hypersensitivity. *(750)*

    a. _host response to allergen_

    b. _exposure amount_

    c. _nature of the allergen_

    d. _rate of allergen entry_

    e. _repeated exposure_

15. List 14 items in the health care environment that could contain latex. *(746)* _gloves, bananas, avocados, kiwi fruit, tomatoes, water chestnuts, peaches, grapes, apricots. → B/P cuffs, stethoscopes, tourniquets, IV tubing, syringes, electrode pads, O₂ masks, tracheal tubes, colostomy & ileal tubes pouches, urinary catheter, anesthetic masks, adhesive tape._

MULTIPLE CHOICE

Directions: Select the best answer(s) for each of the following questions.

16. In caring for an older adult, what instructions would the nurse give to the UAP that address changes related to aging for the immune system? (Select all that apply.) *(741, 742)*
    1. Promptly assist with toileting to prevent urinary stasis.
    2. Increase fluids (unless contraindicated) to thin secretions.
    3. Apply a thin layer of lotion after bathing to prevent dry skin.
    4. Watch for elevated temperature associated with serious infection.
    5. Perform scrupulous hand hygiene and don clean gloves.
    6. Offer frequent oral hygiene because of decreased saliva production.

17. What is the theory behind progressively increasing the doses of the allergens during perennial immunotherapy? *(742)* *(year round)*
    1. Inhibits the release of leukotrienes and reduces allergic symptoms
    2. Allows the individual to build up a tolerance without having symptoms
    3. Competes with histamine by attaching to the cell surface receptors
    4. Inhibits further release of chemical mediators from mast cells

18. If medications are administered in error to a patient who is hypersensitive, which route will produce the most rapid allergic reaction? *(743)*
    1. Oral
    2. Transdermal
    3. Intravenous
    4. Topical

19. The nurse and a friend are ordering lunch. The friend takes 50 mg of diphenhydramine (Benadryl) and then orders oysters, saying, "I'm allergic to oysters, but I just love them, so I take Benadryl." What should the nurse say? *(743)*
    1. "Do you have your cell phone, so we can call 911?"
    2. "Every time you eat oysters, the reaction will get worse."
    3. "You are an adult and you can make your own choices."
    4. "If I have to resuscitate you, I am not going to be happy."

20. The nurse is trying to do an environmental assessment for an elderly patient who is having continuous allergic reactions, but the patient vaguely rambles on about pets, dust, a broken vacuum cleaner, and mold. What is the best intervention to use for this patient? *(743)*
    1. Use simplified and focused yes-or-no questions.
    2. Make an environmental checklist for the patient.
    3. Obtain information from a close relative.
    4. Obtain an order for a home health nurse visit.

21. Within 15 minutes of initiating a blood transfusion, the patient reports shortness of breath, chills, and urticaria. After stopping the transfusion and notifying the health care provider, which laboratory test must be completed? *(748)* *Hives*
    1. Urinalysis
    2. Electrolytes
    3. Platelet count
    4. White blood cell count

22. The suppressed humoral immune response in older adults is associated with: *(749)*
    1. degeneration of the spleen.
    2. decreased production of white blood cells.
    3. reduction in effectiveness of white blood cells.
    4. decreased immunoglobulin levels.

23. During plasmapheresis, the plasma may be replaced with which of the following? (Select all that apply.) *(749, 750)*
    1. Normal saline
    2. Lactated Ringer's solution
    3. Albumin
    4. 10% dextrose
    5. Fresh-frozen plasma
    6. Dextrose 5% and half normal saline

    Plasma protein freezers

24. The nurse gives a patient his immunotherapy injection and immediately he demonstrates wheezes, impaired breathing, and hypotension. The nurse initiates the anaphylaxis protocol. What is the nurse's first action? *(745)*
    1. Establish an IV to administer 1:10,000 epinephrine hydrochloride.
    2. Adminster 1:1000 epinephrine hydrochloride subcutaneously.
    3. Prepare the equipment and assist the provider to intubate the patient.
    4. Administer a 50-mg oral dose of diphenhydramine (Benadryl).

25. What are examples of passive immunity? (Select all that apply.) *(740)*
    1. Mother breastfeeds her baby
    2. Antivenom given after a snakebite
    3. Immunoglobulin administered postexposure
    4. Child gets hepatitis B vaccine - *Active*
    5. Patient reports having measles during childhood

26. In caring for a patient who recently had an organ transplant, which instructions would the nurse give to the UAP to protect this immunosuppressed patient? *(748)*
    1. The most dangerous period is 7 to 10 days after the transplant.
    2. Remind visitors to check at the nurses' station before entering.
    3. If you are pregnant, the patient's chemotherapy may harm the baby.
    4. If you have a cough or skin infection, don a mask and gown. *Do not allow*

27. The nurse is caring for a patient who underwent plasmapheresis. What is the most important assessment to make after the procedure? *(750)*
    1. Monitor intake and output.
    2. Check blood pressure. *HoTN*
    3. Assess mental status.
    4. Evaluate pain.

    Most common complications —
    HoTN
    citrate Toxicity —
    Ls Anticoagulant.

CRITICAL THINKING ACTIVITIES

Activity 1

28. A 22-year-old patient has just completed allergy testing. Her health care provider has prescribed a regimen of weekly allergy shots. *(742)*

    a.   What special precautions should be taken with the patient after the injection? _____

    _____

    _____

    b.   What teaching should be provided for a patient who is receiving allergy shots at home? _____

    _____

    _____

    _____

    c.   After administering the shots at home for more than a month, the patient calls and reports she has been ill and unable to take the medications for the past 2 weeks. How should the nurse advise the patient?

    _____

    _____

Activity 2

29. A 67-year-old patient voices concern about his health status. He reports he never used to "get sick," but now has been hospitalized three times in the last month with a variety of illnesses. *(742)*

    a.   Discuss how aging affects the immune system. _____

    _____

    _____

    _____

    b.   What should the nurse recommend for measures related to preventing immune disorders in an older patient?

    _____

    _____

    _____

Activity 3

30. Design actual questions that the nurse could use to take a detailed history about a rash to help the health care provider diagnose the patient's allergies. Include: (1) onset, nature, and progression of signs and symptoms; (2) aggravating and alleviating factors; and (3) frequency and duration of signs and symptoms. Assess environmental, household, and occupational factors. *(743)*

_____

_____

_____

_____

_____

_____

_____

_____

_____

_____

_____

_____

Care of the Patient with HIV/AIDS

Answer Key: Textbook page references are provided as a guide for answering these questions. A complete Answer Key is provided in your Additional Learning Resources on Evolve.

MATCHING

Nutritional Management: HIV Infection

Directions: Match the condition associated with HIV infection with the recommended dietary therapy. Indicate your answers in the spaces provided. (779)

Condition

_____ 1. fatigue

_____ 2. anemia

_____ 3. altered taste

_____ 4. fever

_____ 5. candidiasis

_____ 6. nausea and vomiting

_____ 7. diarrhea

_____ 8. constipation

Dietary Recommendation

a. High-calorie, high-protein foods
b. Soft or puréed foods
c. High-calorie foods
d. Diet as tolerated
e. High-iron foods
f. High-fiber foods
g. Lactose-free, low-fat, low-fiber, and high-potassium foods
h. Low-fat foods

TRUE OR FALSE

Directions: Write T for true or F for false in the blanks provided.

_____ 9. Studies have shown that in communities where needle-exchange programs have been established, drug use does not increase and rates of HIV infection are controlled. *(786)*

_____ 10. HIV can only be transmitted via contaminated equipment used for illicit drugs such as heroin or cocaine. *(784)*

_____ 11. It is impossible to contract HIV by receiving a blood product due to current testing used to detect HIV in donated blood. *(757)*

_____ 12. HIV is classified as "slow" retrovirus or a lentevirus. After infection with these types of viruses, a long time passes before specific signs and symptoms appear. *(759)*

_____ 13. For patients with end-stage HIV disease who undergo palliative care, the focus will be to relieve pain and give emotional support; intravenous therapy, blood transfusions, and antibiotic usage would not be considered. *(774)*

_____ 14. The CDC's recommendations state that informed consent is not needed for HIV testing, but nurses should be aware that state law may require informed consent before drawing blood to test for HIV. *(783)*

TABLE ACTIVITY

15. Directions: In the table below, add the signs and symptoms that the nurse will see in primary HIV infection (acute illness) and signs and symptoms that appear in early HIV disease (symptomatic infection). *(762)*

Primary HIV infection (acute illness)	Early HIV disease (symptomatic infection)

MULTIPLE CHOICE

Directions: Select the best answer(s) for each of the following questions.

16. Which behavior combined with viral load status creates the highest risk for contracting HIV? *(784)*
    1. Infected partner in mid-stage HIV performs insertive oral intercourse.
    2. Uninfected partner receives anal intercourse from infected partner in primary stage.
    3. Infected partner in mid-stage receives vaginal intercourse from uninfected partner.
    4. Uninfected partner performs insertive oral intercourse on infected partner in late stage.

17. What factors increase the risk of HIV for intravenous drug users? (Select all that apply.) *(757)*
    1. Poor nutritional status and poor hygiene
    2. Exchanges sexual activity for drugs
    3. Impaired judgment due to illicit drug use
    4. Less likely to use condoms during sex
    5. Has ready access to sterile equipment
    6. Routinely uses "booting" during injection

18. Which health care worker has sustained the greatest risk for HIV after being exposed to body fluids from patients who are HIV-positive? *(758)*
    1. Deep puncture with a hollow-bore needle filled with blood from a patient's vein
    2. Splashed in the face with saliva and mucus during oral suctioning and hygiene
    3. Glove tears while cleaning the perianal area of a patient who has postpartum bleeding
    4. Patient vomits copious amounts of bloody fluid over the front of the worker's uniform

19. For a health care worker who must take post-exposure antiviral therapy, which signs/symptoms suggest that the worker is developing the most likely adverse effect of the drug therapy? *(758)*
    1. Fatigue, activity intolerance, and a low red blood cell count
    2. Decreased urine output and elevated blood urea nitrogen
    3. Jaundice, malaise, and abnormal liver function tests
    4. Chest pain, arrhythmias, and elevated troponin levels

20. Perinatal or vertical transmission has been reduced by initiating which combination of interventions? *(759)*
    1. Breastfeeding, enhanced maternal nutrition, and voluntary HIV testing
    2. Bottle-feeding, antiretroviral therapy for HIV-infected mothers, and cesarean birth
    3. Early prenatal care, natural childbirth, and antiretroviral therapy for HIV-infected babies
    4. Inducing labor during mid-stage HIV, and giving zidovudine syrup to neonate at birth

21. For a CD$_4^+$ lymphocyte level of 200 cells/mm^3, which clinical manifestations are most likely to be observed? *(762)*
    1. Generally asymptomatic
    2. Mild flulike symptoms
    3. Opportunistic infections
    4. Fatal respiratory complications

22. What differentiates typical progressors from long-term nonprogressors and rapid progressors? *(762)*
    1. Their physiologic response to standard antiviral therapy
    2. The age of the patient (i.e., rapid progressors are usually older)
    3. The length of time between seroconversion and symptom onset
    4. The number and combination of risk factors at time of exposure

23. The patient is advised to be tested for viral load 4 to 6 months after exposure. What is the clinical significance of having a lower viral set point at this stage? *(762)*
    1. Used to determine the risk for exposing partner to HIV
    2. Predicts minor transient respiratory or skin infections
    3. Helps to determine the type and timing of therapy
    4. Used as a predictor for long-term survival

24. A 32-year-old patient diagnosed with HIV reports she is looking into some alternative and complementary therapies to treat her disease. What is the best response? *(769)*
    1. "You should only rely on prescribed medications. "
    2. "Those therapies can be costly and ineffective."
    3. "What kind of therapies are you considering?"
    4. "Let me know how they work for you."

25. While caring for a known HIV-positive patient in the emergency department, the nurse notices the phlebotomist preparing to draw blood. Which nursing action is correct? *(775)*
    1. Do nothing, because all patients should be treated with Standard Precautions.
    2. Ask the technician if the nurse can see him before he starts the procedure.
    3. Flag the chart to let all health care professionals know the patient's status.
    4. Discretely hand a second pair of gloves to the technician as a signal.

26. An HIV-positive patient voices concern about his recurring bouts of diarrhea, because he is making every effort to follow the treatment plan. What factors contribute to the diarrhea? (Select all that apply.) *(776)*
    1. Side effects of the medications
    2. Infections of the gastrointestinal tract
    3. Damage to the intestinal villi
    4. Malabsorption in the intestinal tract
    5. Insufficient personal hygiene

27. A 34-year-old patient has recently been diagnosed with HIV-associated cognitive motor complex. Which assessment will the nurse initiate? *(780)*
    1. Presence of numbness or tingling in hands or feet
    2. Level of consciousness based on Glasgow coma scale
    3. Home safety assessment to identify obstacles in hallways
    4. Pain in the extremities when ambulating or bending

28. The nurse is talking to a 17-year-old sexually active adolescent who is reluctant to use condoms because "It just doesn't feel as good." Which barrier to prevention is the adolescent demonstrating? *(783, 784)*
    1. Denial of risk
    2. Fear of alienation
    3. Lack of access
    4. Anxiety about sex

29. Which sexual activity would be considered the safest? *(784)*
    1. Mutual monogamy
    2. Mutual masturbation
    3. Vaginal sex with condom
    4. Serial monogamy

CRITICAL THINKING ACTIVITIES

Activity 1

30. A nursing student has just been stuck by a needle while providing care for a patient whose lifestyle has placed him at high risk for HIV infection. After reporting to the clinic, she has questions. *(786)*

    a. What course of action should be taken initially? _____

    _____

    _____

    _____

    _____

    b. What patient-based factors will affect her level of susceptibility? _____

    _____

    _____

    _____

    _____

    c. Upon hearing the recommendation for her to begin prophylactic drug therapy, she asks to wait a few days before beginning the medication regimen. How would you advise her?

    _____

    _____

    _____

    _____

d. After a discussion of the need to begin the medications as soon as possible, she asks for an explanation concerning the pros and cons of taking the drugs.

_____

_____

_____

_____

e. The student voices concerns about having contact with her husband and child. How will the nurse respond to her concerns?

_____

_____

_____

_____

Activity 2

31. A commercial sex worker has used the clinic for treatment for sexually transmitted diseases over the past 3 years, but had always declined testing for HIV. Recently, the worker came in more frequently for a variety of infections that never seemed to fully resolve. Several nurses and health care providers talked to this patient about HIV testing and the benefits of early detection, but the patient said she assumes a "don't know, don't tell" position and that she tries to get all of her customers to use condoms. Several months later, the worker is admitted to the hospital for treatment of opportunistic infection secondary to HIV disease. Discuss the legal and ethical dilemmas for the clinic staff. (786, 787)

_____

_____

_____

_____

_____

_____

_____

_____

_____

_____

Activity 3

32. Think about your personal feelings and concerns about taking care of a patient with HIV or AIDS. If possible, interview a nurse (or a patient) who experienced the early days of the HIV epidemic. Compare and contrast your own personal feelings to those of people who experienced the early days of HIV disease.

_____

_____

_____

_____

_____

_____

_____

_____

_____

_____

Care of the Patient with Cancer

Answer Key: Textbook page references are provided as a guide for answering these questions. A complete Answer Key is provided in your Additional Learning Resources on Evolve.

MATCHING

Directions: Match the terms to the correct definition. Indicate your answers in the spaces provided.

Terms

_____   1.   alopecia *(806)*

_____   2.   autologous *(809)*

_____   3.   benign *(796)*

_____   4.   biopsy *(797)*

_____   5.   cachexia *(810)*

_____   6.   carcinogen *(791)*

_____   7.   carcinoma *(796)*

_____   8.   immunosurveillance *(796)*

_____   9.   dysgeusia *(811)*

_____   10. leukopenia *(803)*

_____   11. malignant *(796)*

_____   12. metastasis *(796)*

_____   13. neoplasm *(800)*

_____   14. palliative *(800)*

_____   15. stomatitis *(806)*

_____   16. sarcoma *(796)*

_____   17. thrombocytopenia *(805)*

Definition

a. Malignant tumors

b. Malnutrition, marked by weakness and emaciation

c. Loss of hair due to the destruction of hair follicles

d. Removal of a small piece of living tissue

e. Origin within an individual

f. Change in taste

g. Not recurrent or progressive; nonmalignant

h. Substances known to increase the risk for developing cancer

i. Immune system's recognition and destruction of newly developed abnormal cells

j. Process by which tumor cells spread

k. Reduction in the number of circulating white blood cells

l. Therapy to relieve uncomfortable symptoms, but does not produce a cure

m. Abnormal cell growth with a loss of normal role and function and ability to spread to other body sites

n. Reduction in the number of circulating platelets

o. Uncontrolled or abnormal growth of cells

p. Malignant tumors of connective tissues

q. Inflamed, sore, ulcerated areas developing within the patient's mouth

SHORT ANSWER

18. What are four quality-of-life factors that affect cancer patients and their families? *(812)*

    a. _____

    b. _____

    c. _____

    d. _____

19. Name five common concerns voiced by cancer patients. *(812)*

    a. _____

    b. _____

    c. _____

    d. _____

    e. _____

20. What are the leading primary cancer sites for men? *(790)*

    a. _____

    b. _____

    c. _____

    d. _____

21. What are the leading primary cancer sites for women? *(790)*

    a. _____

    b. _____

    c. _____

    d. _____

22. What are cancer's seven warning signals? *(795)*

    a. _____

    b. _____

    c. _____

    d. _____

    e. _____

    f. _____

    g. _____

TRUE OR FALSE

Directions: Write T for true or F for false in the blanks provided.

_____ 23. The American Cancer Society indicates that in the United States, one out of every two men will develop cancer in their lifetime. *(790)*

_____ 24. Cancer incidence is higher in African Americans than in any other race. *(791)*

_____ 25. If a female has genes *BRCA1* or *BRCA2*, she has a 25% risk of having breast cancer during her lifetime. *(793)*

_____ 26. Cancer cells are not subject to the usual restrictions placed on cell proliferation by the host. *(796)*

FIGURE LABELING

27. Directions: On the figure below, identify the four types of biopsy depicted. *(798)*

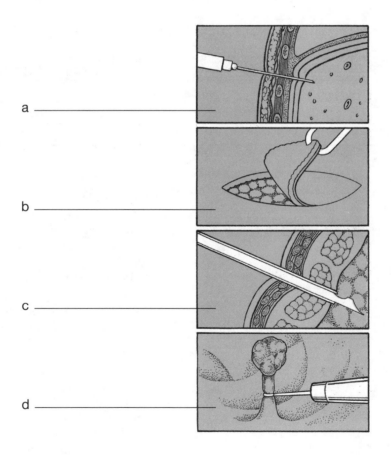

a _____

b _____

c _____

d _____

CLINICAL APPLICATION OF MATH

28. The American Cancer Society recommends adults engage in at least 150 minutes of moderate physical activity each week or 75 minutes of vigorous activity each week. *(795)*
    a. Patient A desires to exercise five times a week doing moderate physical exercise. How many minutes per day will the patient have to spend for each session? _____ min
    b. Patient B desires to exercise six times a week doing moderate physical exercise. How many minutes per day will the patient have to spend for each session? _____ min
    c. Patient C desires to exercise three times a week doing vigorous physical exercise. How many minutes per day will the patient have to spend for each session?_____ min
    d. Patient D desires to exercise seven times a week doing vigorous physical exercise. How many minutes per day will the patient have to spend for each session?_____ min

29. The nurse knows that a 5% weight loss places the patient at risk for malnutrition and the health care provider should be notified. If the patient weighs 140 pounds, how many pounds would be considered a 5% loss? _____ pounds *(811)*

TABLE ACTIVITY

30. Directions: Fill in the normal values in the table below. *(805)*

	Male	**Female**
Erythrocytes (RBCs)	million/mm^3	million/mm^3
Hemoglobin	g/dL	g/dL
Hematocrit	%	%

MULTIPLE CHOICE

Directions: Select the best answer(s) for each of the following questions.

31. What is the single most important lifestyle modification that can reduce risk for cancer? *(791)*
    1. Eat a low-fat, high-fiber diet.
    2. Stop smoking.
    3. Avoid excessive sun exposure.
    4. Limit alcohol consumption.

32. Which dietary recommendation to decrease risk for cancer comes from the National Cancer Institute? *(792)*
    1. Eat four to five servings of lean protein each day.
    2. Eat at least two servings of yellow cheese each day.
    3. Add several types of beans to your diet every week.
    4. Eat at least five servings of fruit and vegetables each day.

33. The patient states that she knows vitamin C is an important nutrient in the prevention of cancer, but she really dislikes citrus fruits. What is the best alternative source that the nurse could suggest? *(792)*
    1. Taking a vitamin C supplement
    2. Trying citrus juice in place of fruit
    3. Eating strawberries or tomatoes
    4. Eating carrots or cauliflower

34. The nurse is talking to a 23-year-old woman about breast self-examination (BSE). What does the nurse tell the patient about timing and frequency of doing BSE? *(795)*
    1. Perform the examination monthly on the first day of your menses.
    2. Perform the examination on the first day of every month.
    3. Perform the examination if you notice a discharge from the nipple.
    4. Perform the examination 2 to 3 days after your period ends.

35. A prostate-specific antigen (PSA) test is usually recommended at age 50. Beginning at age 40, members of which ethnic group need to be advised to get the test? *(800)*
    1. Asian American
    2. African American
    3. Native American
    4. Caucasian American

36. According to clinical staging classification, which stage indicates the most extensive cancer with the poorest prognosis? *(797)*
    1. Stage 0
    2. Stage I
    3. Stage III
    4. Stage IV

37. According to the TNM classification system, which set of parameters suggests the best prognosis? *(797)*
    1. $T_{0;} N_{0;} M_0$
    2. $T_{x;} N_{x;} M_x$
    3. $T_{is;} N_{1;} M_1$
    4. $T_{4;} N_{4;} M_4$

38. The patient is having a radioisotope bone scan. He has had the radioactive material injected into his arm and the nurse encourages him to drink water for the next several hours. What is the purpose of encouraging fluids? *(798)*
    1. Radioisotope that is not picked up by the bone will be flushed through the kidneys.
    2. The radioactive material could be harmful to the kidneys if not diluted and voided.
    3. The fluid enhances the contrast media and facilitates visualization of tumor areas.
    4. Extra fluid thins secretions and improves the visualization of the lung fields.

39. The health care provider is considering magnetic resonance imaging (MRI) for a patient who might have a spinal tumor. Prior to the MRI, the nurse would notify the provider if the patient disclosed which information? *(799)*
    1. History of depression
    2. Family history of breast cancer
    3. History of hip fracture
    4. History of deep vein thrombosis

40. The health care provider informs the nurse that the patient may have metastasis to the bone. The provider requests that the nurse notify him immediately with the relevant results. Which test will the nurse be watching for? *(799)*
    1. Serum calcitonin
    2. Alkaline phosphatase
    3. Carcinomaembryonic antigen
    4. CA-125

41. The patient has a positive guaiac test, but he tells the nurse that he may have not followed the dietary instructions correctly. Which food substance is most likely to cause a false positive? *(800)*
    1. A rare hamburger
    2. A double fudge sundae
    3. French fries with catsup
    4. Caffeinated soda

42. The nurse is present when the health care provider tells the patient that a combination of surgery, radiation, and chemotherapy are needed to treat his cancer. Afterwards, the patient angrily says, "I'm not going to spend my last days getting poked by that doctor. I'm leaving the hospital!" What should the nurse say? *(811)*
    1. "I respect your decision, but is there anything I can do to help?"
    2. "Don't be hasty, you have just had bad news; wait for a while."
    3. "Please don't leave. The doctor is just trying to help you."
    4. "You are upset; that's understandable. Let me call your doctor."

43. The nurse is giving instructions to the UAP on how to assist with hygiene for a patient who is currently undergoing external radiation over a large portion of the trunk. What will the nurse say? *(802)*
    1. Gently clean the skin with a mild soap and flush with warm water.
    2. Do not put lotion, cream, or body powder over the marked areas.
    3. Help the patient take a shower, but use tepid water and a soft cloth.
    4. Shower according to usual procedure, but don't scrub the skin.

44. In caring for the patient who is being treated with internal radiation, what is the most important part of the nursing process for the nurse to prevent self-exposure? *(802)*
    1. Assessment
    2. Planning
    3. Implementation
    4. Evaluation

45. The nurse is instructing the UAP on how to assist the patient who received an applicator of radioactive material in the vagina. What instructions should the nurse give? *(802)*
    1. Spend a maximum of 10 minutes to help with a bed bath from the waist up.
    2. Assist the patient with perineal care because vaginal discharge is likely.
    3. Help the patient ambulate to the shower if she is feeling well enough to walk.
    4. Turn the patient every 2 hours and remind her to do range-of-motion for her arms.

46. The patient is placed on neutropenic precautions for a neutrophil count of fewer than $1000/mm^3$. Which order would the nurse question? *(804)*
    1. Take vital signs every 4 hours.
    2. Report temperature > 100.4° F (38° C).
    3. Catheterize for urine specimen.
    4. Administer filgrastim (Neupogen).

47. The patient has stomatitis secondary to chemotherapy. Which intervention will the nurse use? *(804)*
    1. Suggest that the patient suck hard candy or chew gum.
    2. Help the patient rinse with mouthwash every 2 to 4 hours.
    3. Use a sponge-tipped applicator to perform frequent mouth care.
    4. Suggest drinking warm soup, tea, or other hot liquids.

48. The patient is receiving epoetin alfa (Epogen). Which laboratory finding indicates that the therapy is helping? *(805)*
    1. Normalization of the white cell count
    2. Improvement of the red cell count
    3. Increase in the platelet count
    4. Normalization of the electrolytes

49. Which observation would be consistent with a platelet count of fewer than $20,000/mm^3$? *(805)*
    1. Extreme fatigue
    2. Decreased urine output
    3. High fever
    4. Bleeding gums

50. While caring for a 23-year-old patient undergoing chemotherapy, the patient voices concerns about her hair loss. The nurse advises her that: *(806)*
    1. the loss of her hair will not be permanent.
    2. hair loss will only affect facial areas.
    3. the hair just stops growing temporarily.
    4. when the hair grows back, it will be thicker.

51. During meal planning for a cancer patient, the patient reports that things have a "strange" taste, which is affecting her appetite. Select those possible responses that accurately pertain to her concern. (Select all that apply.) *(811)*
    1. This is a common occurrence and will get better after her treatments end.
    2. This phenomenon is a permanent and unfortunate consequence associated with cancer.
    3. Onion and ham may help to improve the taste of her vegetables.
    4. Lemon juice is frequently used with success to mask these taste alterations.
    5. Eat anything that you feel like, just to keep up your caloric intake.

52. Select those factors shown to have an impact on the determination of how well a patient will cope with a diagnosis of cancer. (Select all that apply.) *(812)*
    1. Age at the time of the diagnosis
    2. Availability of significant others
    3. Presence of symptoms
    4. Socioeconomic status
    5. Gender
    6. Ability to express feelings

53. The nurse is reviewing the patient's medication list and sees that the patient is taking ondansetron (Zofran). What additional intervention will the nurse plan to use? *(806)*
    1. Minimize food odors or noxious smells.
    2. Help the patient dangle before walking.
    3. Check the pulse before giving the drug.
    4. Place a sign on the door to limit visitors.

54. What is an early sign/symptom of tumor lysis syndrome? *(808)*
    1. Anuria
    2. Muscle weakness
    3. Paresthesias
    4. Tetany

55. What is the most effective regimen to manage the patient's cancer pain? *(810)*
    1. Patient-controlled analgesia
    2. Bolus dose for breakthrough pain
    3. Round-the-clock, fixed dose
    4. PRN, based on assessment

CRITICAL THINKING ACTIVITIES

Activity 1

56. During a routine checkup, a 40-year-old man voices questions about his potential for developing colon cancer. He relates his concerns about the recent death of his maternal grandfather from colon cancer. *(792, 793, 800)*

    a. Discuss how a family history of colon cancer affects the recommendations for screening examinations for this patient.

    _____

    _____

    _____

    _____

    b. What preventive behaviors should be included in discussions with this patient? _____

    _____

    _____

    _____

    _____

Activity 2

57. A 32-year-old patient is undergoing radiation therapy for treatment of cervical cancer. *(801-803)*

    a. The patient's mother asks for clarification concerning the differences between radiation therapy and chemotherapy.

    _____

    _____

    _____

    _____

b. After returning to her room after the first treatment, the patient asks if she can shower. Discuss this patient's request.

_____

_____

_____

_____

c. What precautions should be observed with this patient? _____

_____

_____

_____

_____

d. The patient's husband asks about the visitation policy for the couple's 2-year-old daughter. How should the nurse respond?

_____

_____

_____

_____

e. Identify nursing interventions for the care of this patient. _____

_____

_____

_____

_____

_____

_____

_____